Menopause

A self-help guide to feeling better

Wendy Green

Foreword by Janet Brockie, menopause nurse specialist,
John Radcliffe Hospital, Oxford

PERSONAL HEALTH GUIDES

MENOPAUSE: A SELF-HELP GUIDE TO FEELING BETTER

First published in 2009 as *50 Things You Can Do Today to Manage Menopause*
Reprinted 2010, 2013
This edition copyright © Wendy Green, 2016

Vie Books is an imprint of Summersdale Publishers Ltd

Summersdale Publishers Ltd
46 West Street
Chichester
West Sussex
PO19 1RP
UK

www.summersdale.com

Printed and bound by CPI Group (UK) Ltd, Croydon, CR0 4YY

ISBN: 978-1-84953-823-7

612.665

Substantial discounts on bulk quantities of Summersdale books are available to corporations, professional associations and other organisations. For details contact Nicky Douglas by telephone: +44 (0) 1243 756902, fax: +44 (0) 1243 786300 or email: nicky@summersdale.com.

Disclaimer
Every effort has been made to ensure that the information in this book is accurate and current at the time of publication. The author and the publisher cannot accept responsibility for any misuse or misunderstanding of any information contained herein, or any loss, damage or injury, be it health, financial or otherwise, suffered by any individual or group acting upon or relying on information contained herein. None of the opinions or suggestions in this book is intended to replace medical opinion. If you have concerns about your health, please seek professional advice.

To my husband, Gordon — thanks for being so supportive

Acknowledgements

I'd like to thank Janet Brockie, menopause nurse specialist at the John Radcliffe Hospital, Oxford, for her expert advice – particularly regarding HRT – and also for her insight into the issues that can affect women's experiences of the menopause.

I'd also like to thank Jennifer Barclay for commissioning the original book and Claire Plimmer for commissioning this edition. I'm also grateful to Lucy York, Laura Booth, Robert Drew and Sophie Martin for their very helpful editorial input.

Contents

Author's Note...9

Foreword by Janet Brockie, menopause nurse specialist,
John Radcliffe Hospital, Oxford......................................11

Introduction...13

Chapter 1 – Mind Over Menopause............................19
1.   Think positively...20
2.   Take time for things you enjoy............................25
3.   Beat the blues..26
4.   Turn to others for help.......................................29
5.   Manage your stress levels...................................30
6.   Meditate...32
7.   Laugh it off...32
8.   Practise mindfulness...33
9.   Reconnect with nature..33
10. Stroll away stress...34
11. Assert yourself...34
12. Use your brain..35

Chapter 2 – Beat the Heat.......................................37
13. Identify your hot flush triggers...........................38
14. Moderate your alcohol intake.............................39
15. Cut the coffee..40

16. Spare the spices..40
17. Watch your weight..40
18. Eat to beat flushing...41
19. Cool off...41
20. Chill out..42
21. Get moving..43
22. Stop smoking...43
23. Dress appropriately...44
24. Take control of the temperature...........................44
25. Sleep tight..44
26. Don't be embarrassed..45

Chapter 3 – To HRT, or Not to HRT?.............................47
27. Consider whether to use HRT................................47

Chapter 4 – Natural HRT...59
28. Balance your hormones with phytoestrogens..............60
29. Eat foods that lift your mood................................70
30. Boost your memory..72
31. Reduce symptoms with vitamin E
    and unsaturated fats..74
32. Keep your bones healthy......................................77
33. Eat to ease cystitis..82
34. Seek help from herbs...84
35. Take supplements...93

Chapter 5 – More Hints for a Healthier Menopause.......97
36. Walk your way to health.......................................98
37. Be breast aware...100
38. Manage migraines..102

39. Stop cystitis..103
40. Beat incontinence..104
41. Sleep more soundly...105

Chapter 6 – DIY Complementary Therapies................109
42. Apply acupressure..110
43. Use aroma power..111
44. Use flower power..114
45. Get homeopathic healing...................................115
46. Find relief in reflexology....................................117
47. Say 'yes' to yoga...119

Chapter 7 – Look Younger.......................................121
48. Take steps towards younger-looking skin................122
49. Get heavenly hair..132
50. Banish middle-age spread....................................135

Recipes...145

Jargon Buster...153

Useful Products..157

Helpful Books...161

Directory..163

Author's Note

Before I went through the menopause I had a pretty negative view of what it would be like, based on what I'd read in magazines and newspapers and heard from family members, friends and acquaintances. What with feelings of loss, wrinkles, mood swings, hot flushes and broken sleep, there seemed to be little to look forward to!

However, once I learned that a gynaecological condition I had would improve after the menopause, my attitude altered and I began thinking that it could be a positive experience after all. When the menopause came I relied, and still do, on a healthy lifestyle, herbal supplements and a positive outlook to get me through it – though I realise this might not be enough for every woman.

I've found life postmenopause rewarding and exciting, though there have been some health issues to overcome – including chronic migraine and arthritis. The perimenopause and postmenopause can be a bit of a roller coaster ride – especially if you don't quite know what to expect, or what choices you have in dealing with it. I wrote this book to offer easily accessible information about the menopause, HRT and as many self-help options as possible, to enable readers to make sensible choices and find solutions that work for them.

Wendy Green

Foreword

In a world of inequality, the menopause unites all women regardless of race, religion, wealth or education. However, each woman's experience of the menopause is individual, varied and unpredictable. Many women reach the menopause with a personal preference about which treatment options or natural approaches are acceptable for them. But we cannot know beforehand how we will feel or what we will experience.

Attitudes to the menopause vary. In the West, some authors have complained that the menopause is a natural event which has become over-medicalised; alternatively, health care professionals, like myself, may feel that some popular alternative approaches are not supported by sufficient scientific evidence. However, no one has the right to dictate what is the correct course of action for another. Each woman deserves to be able to make an informed decision on what seems correct for her. This book, with its friendly, easy-going style, offers a wide breadth of information and valuable practical advice to meet all needs. It embraces the diversity of women's experiences and responds to their differences.

However they feel about reaching the menopause, women need to be universally encouraged to make the most of this time in their lives, take responsibility for their health and move on with greater confidence to face life's next challenge.

Janet Brockie,
menopause nurse specialist, John Radcliffe Hospital, Oxford

Introduction

What is the menopause?

The literal meaning of the word 'menopause' is 'the last menstrual period', though most women use the term to refer to the years both leading up to and beyond it. The phase leading up to the menopause, when the production of female hormones begins to decline, is actually the perimenopause. The perimenopause can last three to 15 years, but averages between three to six years. The life stage after the menopause is the postmenopause. The age range for most women going through the menopause is between 45 and 55. In some rare cases it can take place as early as the thirties, or as late as 58, but the average age in the UK is 51. Generally, if the menopause occurs before the age of 45 it's classed as premature, though some health professionals would define this as early and menopause before the age of 40 as premature. The age at which you go through the menopause can be inherited, so finding out when your mother had her last menstrual period could give you some idea of when to expect yours. Lifestyle factors are also thought to play a part in the age at which you experience menopause. A stressful life event can trigger early menopause, as can smoking. Other causes include cancer treatments and hysterectomy with, or occasionally without, ovary removal.

Why does it happen?

The female body has a limited supply of eggs and menopause happens when the ovaries run out of eggs and as a result stop producing the female sex hormones oestrogen and progesterone. In one sense it's a non-event, because you will only know for sure that the menopause has happened when you have not had a period in a year. (Only then can you be sure that you're no longer able to get pregnant.)

What are hormones?

Hormones are basically chemical messengers which are released into the bloodstream to affect an organ elsewhere in the body. The hypothalamus at the base of the brain controls menstruation by releasing the hormone gonadotrophin to the pituitary gland. Throughout the reproductive years the pituitary responds by producing two hormones – follicle-stimulating hormone (FSH) and luteinising hormone (LH). These determine the amount of oestrogen and progesterone the ovaries produce. FSH stimulates egg production and LH stimulates ovulation. As you approach menopause you ovulate less, so you can expect erratic/irregular periods until you gradually stop altogether. To compensate, your body releases more FSH and LH, to try to stimulate egg production.

Female hormones

Oestrogen and progesterone are the two main female sex hormones. There are three types of oestrogen – oestradiol, oestrone and oestriol. Oestradiol is the main oestrogen produced by your ovaries. They also produce small amounts of oestrone and continue to do so after the menopause. Your fat cells also convert androstenedione, a male hormone, from the adrenal glands and the ovaries, into oestrone. Oestriol is made in your fat cells, and in the placenta during pregnancy. Oestrogen stimulates the growth of the womb lining, whilst progesterone makes it more nourishing for a fertilised egg.

Oestrogen is responsible for your feminine shape and voice and plays a part in the function of your skin, heart, bones and brain, where it may protect against depression. It's also involved in maintaining your body temperature, which is why many women experience hot flushes when their oestrogen levels drop. For more information about oestrogen and hot flushes, see chapter 2. Progesterone is involved in burning fat for energy, thyroid function and, like oestrogen, is thought to enhance mood and induce calm. Drops in progesterone during the menopause may result in anxiety, depression, irritability, low libido and weight gain. As pregnancy is no longer possible after menopause, your body produces little progesterone – some estimate a mere 120th of the amount produced during your early twenties.

Postmenopausal hormones

Although oestrogen levels drop dramatically after the ovaries stop producing eggs (by up to 60 per cent), this hormone doesn't disappear entirely – the body just finds other ways of producing it. Before the menopause your main oestrogen is oestradiol. After the menopause oestrone becomes your main form of oestrogen.

As the adrenal glands produce androstenedione, which is converted into oestrone, it's important to keep them healthy and functioning well during this time of your life by following a healthy lifestyle and managing stress. Stress management is vital, because the adrenal glands are also responsible for the production of stress hormones. If you're under extreme stress, your adrenal glands may not cope with producing androstenedione as well. Your fat cells convert androstenedione into oestrone, so it's important to avoid being too thin.

Is it the menopause?

Many women start noticing changes in their menstrual cycle without realising their significance. One of the first signs of the perimenopause is your periods becoming irregular due to fluctuating hormone production as the number of eggs released declines. The cycle length may shorten, or you could sometimes miss a period altogether.

Other symptoms caused by these hormonal changes include:

- Period changes – they may get heavier, or lighter

- Mood swings – including anxiety, depression and irritability

- Poor concentration and memory loss – because oestrogen is involved in blood flow to the brain and brain function

- Hot flushes and night sweats – because falling oestrogen levels affect the hypothalamus gland - the body's thermostat

- Low libido – mood swings and insomnia may also contribute to this

- Vaginal dryness – due to thinning and loss of elasticity of skin and tissues

- Increased urgency and frequency of urination – due to bladder losing tone and elasticity leading to a reduced ability to hold urine

- Urine infections – due to bladder and vaginal tissue thinning, making them more susceptible to infection or injury

- Tiredness – due to disturbed sleep and insomnia

- Aches and pains - due to thinning of bones and changes in joint tissues

- Weight gain – especially around the middle – as the body tries to hang on to oestrogen-producing fat cells

- Headaches and migraines – may worsen during perimenopause, but improve postmenopause, when hormone levels stabilise

Individual women suffer from these problems in varying degrees, with a lucky few sailing through virtually problem-free.

Heavy bleeding can occasionally signify something more serious, so if you suffer from unusually heavy, very irregular or painful periods it's probably a good idea to see your GP for a check-up, just to rule out anything more sinister. Any bleeding after the age of 58 should be investigated.

Note

Thyroid disease also presents similar symptoms to the menopause. An underactive thyroid can lead to heat intolerance, fatigue, lethargy, heavy, irregular or prolonged periods, hair loss, dry skin, insomnia, weight gain and cystitis. Signs of an overactive thyroid include weight loss, heat intolerance and increased sweating, infrequent periods and sleep problems. These and other forms of thyroid disease may also lead to swelling of the thyroid gland in the neck. An organisation called Thyroid UK offers information and support – further details are in the directory at the end of the book. If you're in any doubt about the cause of your symptoms, consult your GP, who can perform appropriate tests.

Home tests

If you're experiencing some of these symptoms but want to be sure that they're due to the menopause approaching rather than some other condition, there's a test which measures the level of FSH in your blood to find out roughly what stage you're at. Your GP can do this test for you, or you can do a home test. However, bear in mind that FSH levels can fluctuate, so the test should be done more than once to get a more reliable assessment. There are details of home tests in the Useful Products section.

After the menopause

After the menopause you may continue to suffer from any or all of these symptoms – except, of course, the menstrual bleeding. You're also likely to notice other changes, such as thinning hair and skin. This is because lower levels of oestrogen lead to a reduction of collagen – a sticky protein which basically keeps cells together. Less oestrogen also leads to less calcium and collagen in the bones, making you more at risk of developing osteoporosis (bone loss). Also, oestrogen seems to reduce cholesterol and lipid levels, so after the menopause this benefit is lost, leading to a much bigger risk of heart attack and stroke.

Whilst some of these symptoms are related to hormonal decline, others may simply be due to the ageing process, since men of a similar age also report psychological problems, weight gain and ageing skin and hair. A healthy lifestyle that includes appropriate nutrition, adequate exercise, a positive attitude and stress management has been shown to reduce symptoms and help prevent the onset of the more serious conditions associated with the menopause and beyond, such as cardiovascular disease, breast cancer and osteoporosis. This guide offers information, tips and techniques to enable you to achieve this.

Chapter 1

Mind Over Menopause

Your attitude towards the menopause can have a huge influence on how you cope with it, both physically and mentally. This is clear when you look at how women view the menopause in different cultures. For example, in China the menopause is seen as a natural part of ageing, with women there reporting fewer hot flushes. Seventy per cent of Malaysian women claim not to suffer from hot flushes, and many see the menopause as a blessing. Indian women generally view the menopause as a natural part of ageing, so they don't seek medical help. Kung women in South Africa look forward to the menopause because they enjoy higher status afterwards and don't even have a word for hot flush! These women's different experiences of the menopause may also be due to their different lifestyles – especially in terms of diet. For example, Japanese women consume a lot of soya products, which may explain why they report few menopausal symptoms.

In Westernised countries the menopause has been medicalised and turned into a deficiency disease, rather than a natural process that all women go through. That isn't to say that menopausal symptoms are imagined – most women suffer from at least some of the recognised symptoms to varying degrees. On the other hand, viewing it as an illness that requires treatment isn't helpful either. In Western culture the menopause has traditionally been viewed as a time of loss – the loss of hormones and fertility and often the loss of children as they grow up and leave home. But, back in the early 1990s, Germaine Greer offered a more positive viewpoint when she suggested that postmenopausal women could become the person they were before their lives were taken over by their biological urge to have babies. There now seems to be a growing shift in perspective. As one woman who recently set up a successful business in her fifties aptly put it, 'You get the freedom of your teenage years, but without the spots and nervousness… you get the confidence to make things happen.'

❶ Think positively

Though the menopause can cause some unpleasant symptoms, it's not an illness, but a natural process that all women go through. Focus on the positive aspects of the physical changes, such as freedom from periods and the need for contraception, and remember that all of the symptoms are temporary.

The singer Lulu commented that she'd tried HRT (see chapter 3) for a couple of months and then decided to try the 'alternative medicine route'. She added, 'I get hot flushes, of course, and I become emotional, but it's a kind of sweet thing when things really touch you, you know? It's heartwarming, like the heart opens up.' Perhaps she's lucky enough not to experience severe symptoms, but it may be that her positive attitude towards her life and her symptoms is helping too.

Brain change

According to American psychiatrist Dr Louann Brizendine, declining levels of oestrogen and progesterone affect the way women think before, during and after the menopause. Irregular hormone levels at the perimenopause lead to a corresponding fluctuation in mood, libido and sleep patterns, as well as hot flushes, anxiety and irritability.

The menopause is characterised by low oestrogen levels and little progesterone. Women in this phase, according to Brizendine, concentrate on their health and new challenges. Postmenopausal women have low, but steady, levels of oestrogen and testosterone and low oxytocin – the 'nurturing hormone' – which leaves them calmer, less emotional and less interested in caring for others. As a result, women at this stage may start to focus more on themselves and begin to develop new ideas and ambitions.

Social change

Brizendine's theories help to explain this new attitude to life among women 'of a certain age', but other factors are involved. For a start, female baby boomers – born in the post-war years between 1946 and 1964 – like their male counterparts, view themselves as more like their children than their parents or grandparents ever did. They're healthier and wealthier than previous generations, so they can look forward to a more active old age. They're also more rebellious and anti-establishment than their predecessors and have a reputation for refusing to grow old gracefully!

Feminism and equal opportunities legislation have also vastly increased opportunities for women – little wonder that many postmenopausal women are no longer content to sit at home and grow old. As women's life expectancy increases, many can look forward to living another two or three decades postmenopause. After spending years at home caring for children, many are deciding it's time to make their mark and resurrect their careers. As a result, unlike previous generations, postmenopausal women are financially independent and statistics show they're increasingly leaving husbands whose outlook on life differs vastly from their own.

Positive role models

An increasing number of celebrities aged 50 plus are also refusing to fade quietly into the background. 'Queen of Pop' Madonna, now in her late fifties, looks far younger – thanks to a strict diet and exercise regime. She's currently the highest-earning female singer in the world and her career continues to go from strength to strength. The Scottish singer Lulu, who is in her late sixties, recently spoke of hoping to 'age disgracefully' and shows no sign of slowing down, following the launch of her own skin care range. TV presenter Anne Robinson, who's now in her seventies, and still working, revealed the secrets of her continuing success when she remarked: 'For a woman to have longevity on televison you have got to be clever, versatile, funny – and thin.' Other celebrity role models include Helen Mirren, Joanna Lumley, Jane Seymour and Twiggy, to name but a few.

Build a positive self-image

To reach your goals, you need to believe that you're capable of achieving them. If you've spent the last couple of decades looking after a family and putting their needs before your own, you may find the idea of focussing on your own needs and trying new things a little scary – especially if your self-confidence is low.

What's your self-image like? Do you see yourself as a capable, intelligent and talented human-being, or do you lack the confidence to get what you want from life? Your self-image is based on your self-talk – the ongoing internal conversation you have with yourself. Your self-talk is based on the beliefs and opinions you've formed about yourself as a result of positive and negative experiences and feedback from others.

Positive self-talk leads to a positive self-image, which results in high self-esteem. High self-esteem gives you the confidence to go out and achieve your goals. If your self-talk is negative and you constantly tell yourself 'I can't', 'I'm no good at this', 'I've never been able to...' your actions will reflect the negative self-image your thoughts create. If your self-talk is positive, as in 'I can' or 'I'm good at this', you'll act accordingly. As the life coach Fiona Harrold says in her book, *Be Your Own Life Coach*, 'Believe you can do anything you want and you will.'

Instant self-esteem

Make a list of ten things you've done or do well, e.g. 'I'm a good mother', 'Passing my driving test', 'I'm a fantastic cook', 'I'm brilliant at my job'. It could include the qualifications you've achieved, or positive aspects of your personality – like being thoughtful, or a good listener. In our culture, stating what you're good at is often viewed as boastfulness, so you may feel uncomfortable, but reminding yourself of your achievements and strengths is a sure-fire way of increasing your self-esteem. Whenever self-doubt creeps in, look at your list, or write a new one!

Affirm and achieve

'When you repeat affirmations over and over again,
not only do subtle changes occur within you,
altering the way you act and feel, but the world
reacts to you in a more positive way.'
Susan Jeffers, Ph.D., author

An affirmation is a sentence that states your goal as though you've already achieved it. Repeating your affirmation again and again, until your subconscious mind believes it to be true, enables you to achieve your dreams by changing your self-talk.

An affirmation needs to be personal, so include the word 'I'. It must be positive, so describe what you want to achieve rather than what you don't. Use words that suggest achievement, such as 'I am', 'I have' or 'I do'. How will you feel when you've achieved your goal? Happy? Calm? Excited? Thrilled? Elated? Attaching positive emotions to your goal will make it seem more real and achievable. You'll also see results more quickly. Writing your affirmation as if it's happening now will make it far more effective. Make your affirmation specific: how and when will you achieve it? Finally, make it realistic: can you see yourself achieving it? For example, if your goal is 'to exercise regularly', a good affirmation that incorporates all of these points would be: 'I enjoy walking briskly for half an hour every day, between 6 p.m. and 6.30 p.m. – I feel healthy and energetic.' If your goal is 'to lose weight' your affirmation might be: 'It's Christmas Day – I now weigh 9 stone because I eat healthily, and I love shopping for size 12 clothes.'

Read, see, feel and hear your goal

To fix your affirmation in your subconscious mind, read it first. Then close your eyes and visualise the scene your words paint. Imagine yourself experiencing your goal in detail. Feel the emotions you've linked to your goal. Hear the words your family and friends will use to compliment you when you achieve it. Reading, picturing, feeling and hearing your affirmation has a strong effect on your subconscious mind.

Your subconscious mind can't tell the difference between what happens in reality and what's taken place in your imagination. If you regularly focus on your affirmations, you'll find yourself acting in a way that supports your new self-image. So, if you affirm that you exercise regularly, you'll take more exercise. If you affirm you've lost weight, you'll adopt the diet and exercise habits of a slim person.

2 Take time for things you enjoy

'It is never too late to be what you might have been.'
George Eliot, novelist

Living life to the full isn't just for the privileged few. You can do it too. Avoid the 'empty nest' syndrome if you have children and they leave home by making the most of your new-found freedom. Make the most of the positive physical and psychological changes the menopause brings. Focus on your career. Cultivate new hobbies and interests. View this life stage as a time for personal growth. Do the things you didn't have time for whilst raising your family.

Find your postmenopausal zest

The successful actress Julie Walters said, 'It's a good time of life after the menopause,' adding that once the hot flushes stopped and things settled down again, she found she had more energy and felt emotionally ready to get on with the rest of her life. The anthropologist Margaret Mead called the feeling of rejuvenation many women experience at this time 'postmenopausal zest' – make sure you find yours.

Dare to dream

Deciding what you want to do with your life and setting goals helps you make your dreams a reality. Whether you want to travel the world, learn how to salsa or set up your own business, you first need to identify what you want to achieve.

Think about what you enjoy doing, or would like to try. What were your strengths at school? Is there anything you love doing so much, you'd do it regardless of the financial rewards? Be true to yourself and you'll rediscover what you really want. Imagine leading a life you love, rather than one you feel you should. What job would you do? What would your interests be? What sort of friends would you choose? Use your answers to these questions to help you identify your goals. In her book, *Making the Big Leap*, life coach Suzy Greaves comments, 'To live a different kind of life, you have to start living by your own rules and rediscover what you want for yourself.'

Don't feel guilty about spending time doing the things you love. If you have spent your life putting the needs of others before your own, you may find this hard. But remember: the happier and more fulfilled you are, the nicer you are to be around.

③ Beat the blues

Depression is one of the symptoms linked to the menopause, especially if you view the menopause negatively. You can help lift your depression by adopting a more positive attitude.

Fluctuating hormone levels can have an effect on your mood. Coping with menopausal symptoms such as flushes and insomnia can also contribute, so it's important to deal with these symptoms first.

Depression is often linked to repressed anger about something going on in your life. Just sitting and writing down who, or what, you're angry about often helps. Acknowledging and expressing your anger paves the way for you to work out what you need to do to prevent or deal with similar situations in the future. For example, you may need to practise the assertiveness skills outlined further on in this chapter.

Sometimes depression stems from general unhappiness with a situation in your life. It could be your job, a relationship or some other aspect of your life. By identifying what it is that isn't working and is causing you unhappiness, you can begin to consider the changes you could make to improve things. For example, could you cut the hours you work, or retrain for a new career? Could you breathe new life into your relationship, or is it time to move on? If you're unsure, seeing a Relate counsellor may help you to decide. You can find the contact details for Relate in the directory at the end of the book.

Treat yourself more kindly

To combat the short-term blues, treat yourself more kindly, allow yourself to cry and talk about your feelings to someone you can trust. Do something you enjoy, even if it's just taking a scented bath, reading a novel by your favourite author or playing your favourite music – anything that reminds you that life can be pleasurable will help. Try to follow a healthy lifestyle. In particular, make sure you get out in daylight as much as possible. This will help you avoid suffering from seasonal affective disorder, which is caused by a lack of sunshine and happens largely in the winter months.

It's important to remember that no one is happy all of the time. Unhappiness is an inevitable part of life – according to experts it's only an illness when it lasts longer than a week or two and seriously affects your ability to lead a normal life. This is when you should consider visiting your GP. Supplements such as cod liver oil, St John's wort and 5-HTP have been shown to be effective in treating mild to moderate depression (see chapter 4 for details, plus information on mood-boosting foods).

Happiness booster

Psychologists argue that happiness isn't dependent on material wealth or success; as a nation we are richer than ever – but we aren't any happier. In surveys, fewer people describe themselves as being happy than a few decades ago. It would seem that taking the time to appreciate what we've already got, rather than hankering after the things we don't have, can make us feel instantly happier. So try reminding yourself of at least five things you should be thankful for, every day. Most of us have a lot to be grateful for, but we rarely acknowledge the fact. Family and friends, good health, sufficient food, a nice home… the list is endless!

The Happiness Project

The Happiness Project was formed in 1996 by Dr Robert Holden, an expert in positive psychology, and is based on the idea that happiness is within everyone's reach. The project offers a five-day happiness training course spread across eight weeks. Holden believes that the keys to happiness include self-acceptance, positive self-image and the ability to embrace and understand sadness. (See Directory for more information and contact details.)

4 Turn to others for help

Some women find they have extra responsibilities at the time when they are going through the menopause – they may still help their grown-up children financially, plus the added burdens of caring for grandchildren and elderly, possibly unwell, parents and in-laws. If you're experiencing financial problems, perhaps as a result of assisting other family members financially, being a carer, or unemployment, there are agencies that can help, such as the Citizen's Advice Bureau and the National Debtline. If you feel family demands are impacting on your mental health, consider ways you could share tasks. Are there other family members that could shoulder more responsibility? If you feel uncomfortable about asking others for help, try using the assertiveness techniques mentioned near the end of this chapter.

If others are unable or unwilling to help or there's no one else to turn to, there are organisations that can offer support and advice, such as The Princess Royal Trust for Carers, which can also put you in touch with your nearest support group. Elderly Parents is another organisation that may be able to help with the problems associated with caring for ageing parents. Your local social services offer support and advice to carers, as well as home, day and residential care services. You can contact them to ask for a needs assessment for both yourself and the person you care for.

Social network

Make time to see family and friends regularly. There's evidence that people who have a good social network enjoy better mental health than those who don't, probably because they're more likely to have people they can confide in when they have problems. This is especially important if you live alone.

If you don't have anyone you can confide in, your GP may refer you to a qualified counsellor. The Samaritans are available at any time of day or night to listen to your problems and, if necessary, signpost you to appropriate agencies. Mind also offers various forms of support including counselling, befriending and advocacy. If you've recently been bereaved, Cruse Bereavement Care offers support, information and advice to help you cope with your loss. You can find further information and the contact details for all of the organisations I've mentioned in the directory at the end of this book.

⑤ Manage your stress levels

Stress and anxiety during and after the menopause can increase flushing, insomnia, depression and other symptoms. This may be because they compromise the adrenal glands' ability to produce androstenedione.

Managing your stress levels will help you to control your menopausal symptoms and reduce your risk of suffering from any of the life-threatening conditions associated with the postmenopause.

What is stress?

Stress is the way the mind and body respond to situations and pressures which leave us feeling inadequate, or unable to cope. One person may cope well in a situation that another finds stressful. It depends on the individual's perception of it and their ability to deal with it.

The brain reacts to stress by priming the body to either stay put and face the perceived threat, or to run away (fight or flight). It does this by releasing hormones, including adrenaline, noradrenaline and cortisol, into the bloodstream. These cause the heart rate and breathing patterns to speed up and may induce sweating. Glucose and fatty acid levels in the blood rise to give us the energy to deal with the threat.

Stress and your health

Research shows that over time the chemical effects of stress can increase the risk of high blood pressure, coronary heart disease (CHD), stroke, cancer, obesity, diabetes, depression and even memory loss and fertility problems. Also, if the stressor isn't removed, or managed, cortisol levels stay high. The body adapts to this constant state of emergency by craving high energy, sugary and fatty foods to provide a fat store around the waist, which provides an easily converted energy source. This is the most risky place to store fat because it increases the risk of CHD, stroke and diabetes – especially after the menopause, when a reduction in oestrogen increases CHD risk. For advice on avoiding 'middle-age spread', see chapter 7.

Anxiety is part of the 'fight or flight' reaction to stress. Whilst it's a normal reaction to stressful situations, it becomes a problem when it becomes the normal mindset. It can lead to an inability to relax, panic attacks, palpitations and breathing problems.

Identify and avoid causes of stress

For a week or two, note down situations, times, places and people that lead to you feeling stressed. Once you've identified your stressors, identify ways to avoid or at least minimise them. 'No' is a little word that can reduce your stress levels dramatically. Say 'no' to things you don't have time for, or don't want to do.

6 Meditate

Practise meditation. It's a simple technique which, if practised regularly, has been shown to lower stress hormone levels, ease anxiety, combat tiredness and boost energy and clear thinking. Here's a simple meditation: sit comfortably and close your eyes. Breathe in through your nose deeply and slowly, inflating your stomach. Breathe out slowly and deeply through your mouth, deflating your stomach. Choose a word which suggests calmness to you, e.g. 'calm', 'peace', 'harmony' or 'relax'. Repeat the word over and over in your mind whilst visualising a place or an object that induces calmness in you, for example a river flowing or a candle flickering. Engage your other senses – imagine the sound of the water trickling by, feel the warmth of the candle. Each time your mind wanders, acknowledge it, then re-focus on your chosen image and word. To learn more about meditation techniques go to www.t-m.org.uk.

7 Laugh it off

Laughter really is the best medicine! It seems that a good belly-laugh can reduce the stress hormone cortisol and increase mood-boosting serotonin levels. Recent research suggests that women benefit more from this than men. Women who see the funny side of life enjoy a reduced risk of the health problems associated with the stress hormone cortisol, including high blood pressure, obesity, heart disease and even cancer. Laughing also relaxes the muscles in the upper body and improves the blood supply to organs such as the liver, spleen, pancreas, kidneys and adrenal glands. So make time to watch your favourite comedies and be with people who make you laugh.

8 Practise mindfulness

Mindfulness involves focussing on the present instead of worrying about the past or future and has its roots in Buddhism. It's based on the philosophy that we can't change the past, or predict the future, but we can affect what's happening right now. By living fully in the here and now you can perform to the best of your ability, whereas worrying about the past and future can hamper how you function and increase stress levels unnecessarily. To help you focus more on the present it might be helpful to keep a daily diary.

9 Reconnect with nature

Activities like watching the sea, going for a walk in the park or countryside, or even just sitting in the garden have been shown to reduce heart rate, blood pressure and muscle tension. Experts believe that the higher levels of negative ions near areas with running water, trees and mountains may be partly responsible. Others claim it's due to 'biophilia' – the theory that man has a natural affinity with nature. Studies in the Netherlands and Japan show that people living in or near green areas enjoy a longer life and better health than those who live in urban environments.

> **Have a hug**
> Hugging regularly has been shown to reduce stress hormones in the bloodstream and lower blood pressure.

10 Stroll away stress

Taking a stroll could help you beat stress and stave off depression and anxiety. A recent eight-year US study found that menopausal women who walked five times a week for at least 40 minutes suffered less stress, anxiety and depression than women who were fairly inactive. It's thought walking encourages the brain to release 'feel good hormones', or endorphins. For more information on how walking regularly can help prevent many menopausal symptoms, see chapter 5.

11 Assert yourself

If you often find yourself giving in to others and not expressing your feelings to avoid hurting or upsetting them, or to gain their approval, or if you regularly allow yourself to be manipulated into doing things you don't want to do, perhaps you need to become more assertive. Being assertive means you can say what you want, feel and need calmly and confidently, without being aggressive or causing hurt to others. Try the following techniques to boost your self-assertiveness skills, so that you take control of your life and do things because you want to, rather than simply to appease other people.

- Show ownership of your thoughts, feelings and behaviour by using 'I' rather than 'we', 'you' or 'it'. So rather than 'You make me angry' state 'I feel angry when you...'

- When you have made a choice not to do something, say 'won't' rather than 'can't' to show you've made an active decision.

- Use 'choose to' rather than 'have to' and 'could' rather than 'should' to demonstrate that you always have choice.

- When you feel your needs aren't being listened to, state what you want calmly, repeating it until the other person shows they've taken on board what you've said.

- When making a request, state exactly what you want in a calm, clear, straightforward way. You could begin with 'I would like...', 'I want...' or 'I would appreciate'.

- When refusing a request, speak firmly but calmly, giving the reason why, without apologising. Repeat if necessary.

- When you disagree with someone, say so using the word 'I'. Explain why you disagree, whilst accepting the other person's right to have a different point of view.

12 Use your brain

A survey of 500 menopausal women in 2003 revealed that seven out of ten complained of poor concentration and memory. Falling oestrogen levels, poor sleep patterns and low mood could all contribute.

However, according to many psychologists, declining brain function as we age isn't inevitable. When it comes to brain function, it's a case of either use it or lose it. The more you use your brain, the better it functions. Blood flow is increased and neurons – brain cells that pass on messages – make better connections with other neurons. Lack of use leads to a weaker performance in the different brain areas, including that associated with memory.

Brain gym

Beat the memory and concentration problems associated with the menopause by exercising your mind on a daily basis. Doing puzzles such as crosswords and sudoku, playing Scrabble, or learning something new (for example a foreign language) stimulates and challenges the mind, boosting concentration and helping retain memory. Keeping a diary involves using your memory, as you think back to the day's events. Reading uses both sides of the brain. To enhance your powers of recall, look up any words you don't know the meaning of, then resolve to use them. Learning a poem by heart each week has been shown to improve both short- and long-term memory. Playing a musical instrument can also enhance mental function.

Physical activity improves brain function too. Recent research suggests that, among older people, regular exercise boosts blood flow to the brain, stimulating cell growth and protecting against dementia. Being active also reduces the risk of high blood pressure, which is linked to reduced blood flow to the brain and mental decline. For more ideas on how to increase your physical activity, see 'Get moving' in chapter 2.

Chapter 2

Beat the Heat

Hot flushes, also known as hot flashes, or power surges in the US, are a common symptom of the menopause. Eight out of ten menopausal women in the UK report suffering from hot flushes for at least a year. Some women experience them during the perimenopause, others don't experience them until after the menopause. Around one in three are affected for five years, with one in ten having flushes for up to ten years. Because hormone levels can rise and fall, hot flushes may come and go.

This chapter looks at practical tips that can help you cope with or reduce the flushes you experience. In chapter 4, you'll find nutritional advice that may help to reduce flushing.

What is a hot flush?

A hot flush occurs when there's a sudden dilation (widening) of blood vessels in the skin, which leads to heat being released – perhaps the US term 'hot flash', suggesting something happening quickly, is more apt. Flushing is thought to be linked to falling oestrogen levels causing a hormonal imbalance in the hypothalamus. The hypothalamus is the part of the brain which controls, among other things, the body's temperature regulatory system. The exact mechanism is unknown, but it's thought that these hormonal ebbs and flows can lead to the body's internal thermostat being in a state of flux. Recent research suggests that the brain chemical serotonin and its receptors are somehow implicated. Flushes that occur during the night are usually referred to as night sweats and often disrupt sleep.

What does a flush feel like?

A flush causes a sudden and uncomfortable feeling of extreme heat, which radiates upwards from the chest and back to the neck and face. It can trigger heavy sweating and redness and some women also experience palpitations, dizziness, weakness and anxiety. As the feeling of heat subsides, many women feel cold and clammy, because the sweating mechanism reduces the body's temperature. A flush can last from just a few seconds to 10 minutes, but the average duration is 4 minutes.

13 Identify your hot flush triggers

Anything that can cause the body temperature to go up can act as a trigger for flushing, e.g. an over warm room or hot food and drink. Stress also seems to increase flushing. As noted in chapter 1, this may be due to it interfering with the adrenal glands' ability to produce androstenedione, a precursor to oestrone.

If you suffer from frequent flushes, it may help for you to record when and where they occur and your emotions just beforehand, as well as any foods or drinks you had. You should then be able to identify your triggers and plan ways to avoid or at least minimise them.

For example, do they tend to take place in the morning, during the day or in the evening? Do they come on when you're stressed, tired or upset? Do you get a flush after you've drunk tea or coffee? Do they mainly happen when you go from a cool environment to a warmer one?

Date/time	Location	Emotions prior to flush	Environment – hot/cool	Food/drinks consumed prior to flush

14 Moderate your alcohol intake

A study in 2004 suggested that drinking moderately – up to five alcoholic drinks per week – may reduce the number of hot flushes suffered during the perimenopause by boosting blood oestrogen levels. Conversely, excessive drinking – more than 14 units a week – is linked to an increase in flushes. Research suggests that this may be due to reduced blood oestrogen levels, possibly as a result of the toxic effects of alcohol on the ovaries and liver. Alcohol also relaxes the muscles in the blood vessels, causing them to widen and increasing blood flow and the risk of flushing. A small (125 ml) glass of wine contains, on average, 1.5 units, while a large (175 ml) glass contains two.

15 Cut the coffee

Research suggests that cutting down on the amount of coffee you drink or switching to de-caff can help to reduce hot flushes. The combination of caffeine, which is a stimulant, and the temperature of the drink can trigger hot flushes in many women. This applies to cola and tea as well, though tea contains around only half as much caffeine. Try replacing one or two cuppas a day with plain water, or a herbal tea you enjoy. Most supermarkets now stock a variety of herbal teas. See chapter 4 for details of herbal teas that could help beat flushes.

16 Spare the spices

Monitor your reaction to spicy foods – some women find they can bring on flushes and are best avoided. Use garlic and herbs such as sage, fennel and parsley in cooking instead and you'll also benefit from the phytoestrogens – plant hormones – that they contain.

17 Watch your weight

There's evidence to suggest that being excessively overweight during the perimenopause can trigger flushing, possibly because the extra weight leads to reduced levels of androstenedione, which means less oestrone can be produced in the fat cells. Being too thin may also increase flushing, because fewer fat cells also means less oestrone is produced. Being a healthy weight may mean fewer flushes, because you'll both produce enough androstenedione and have sufficient fat cells in which to store it for conversion into oestrone. To find out whether you're a healthy weight and for advice on weight management, see chapter 7.

18 Eat to beat flushing

Peaks and troughs in your blood sugar levels may also exacerbate flushing. Avoid foods containing refined sugars and carbohydrates such as sweets, chocolate, cakes and biscuits. Eating refined sugar gives you a quick energy boost, which in turn generates heat and can lead to flushing. Instead, opt for slow-burning natural sugars by eating fresh and dried fruits. If you dislike hot drinks without sugar, try using a little honey instead. Honey is thought to raise the blood sugar more slowly than refined sugar. It's best to eat little and often, because digesting large meals can generate heat, which in turn can trigger hot flushes. You should also choose foods with a low glycaemic index, which means they are digested slowly, causing a gradual rise in your blood sugar (see 'Banish middle-aged spread' in chapter 7). Including protein foods such as lean meat and low-fat dairy products in your diet can also help, because they slow down the rate at which glucose is absorbed.

19 Cool off

Try these top tips for instant cooling relief from the effects of a hot flush:

- Running your inner wrists under a cold tap for a minute or 2 can cool you down rapidly.

- When you feel a flush coming on, sip cold water to cool you down and relieve the effects.

- Carry a handbag-sized mineral water spray and spray your face and neck to take the heat out of a flush. Make sure you carry tissues to blot your skin afterwards. Rose water used in the same way is aromatic and cooling.

- Carry a pack of body wipes in your handbag. They're great for freshening up after a hot flush. Lemon or cucumber fragranced ones are particularly cooling and refreshing. For added coolness, store them in the fridge.

- As an alternative to wipes, keep a damp face cloth in the fridge. To enhance the effects, add a few drops of cooling peppermint, or hormone-balancing geranium, clary sage or rose oil to water and wring the cloth out in the solution.

- Place a bag of frozen vegetables from the freezer on your face, neck, inner arms and wrists for instant cooling relief from a hot flush.

- At the office, use a desk fan – even the small, inexpensive models that plug into your computer are surprisingly effective.

20 Chill out

Research suggests that regular relaxation can reduce flushing by up to 60 per cent. For ideas on reducing stress, see chapter 1.

During a flush, relax and take deep, calming breaths rather than tensing up and you may find it passes more quickly. One study suggested that deep breathing can cut the number of flushes experienced by half. Aim to inhale slowly through your nostrils to a count of three whilst expanding your stomach. Hold for a count of three and then exhale through your mouth counting to six, whilst flattening your stomach.

When a flush strikes, visualise being in a cool place – perhaps in an icy cold plunge pool. Imagine a feeling of icy coldness washing over you, from your feet right up to your head.

21 Get moving

Studies show that being physically active for 1 to 3 hours a week reduces the occurrence of hot flushes and night sweats. You don't have to go to the gym – you could just try to be more active in your daily life. Find an activity you enjoy – such as dancing or swimming – rather than something you find a chore, and you're more likely to continue doing it in the long term. That may sound obvious, but many people take up a punishing exercise regime that they don't enjoy and consequently don't sustain. See chapter 5 for ideas on how to achieve this.

22 Stop smoking

Smoking increases your risk of flushing as well as contributing to other menopause-related symptoms and conditions. Giving up is difficult, but there is help available – see your GP for details of your nearest Smoking Cessation clinic, where you'll be offered advice and support. Alternatively, visit www.gosmokefree.nhs.uk or call the free NHS Smoking Helpline on 0800 022 4332 for information about the free NHS services available to help you stop smoking.

23 Dress appropriately

Synthetic fibres such as nylon and polyester can make the sweating that comes with hot flushes worse. Try wearing clothes made from cotton and linen, as they absorb sweat. Go for loose fitting clothes and wear layers; then when you feel yourself heating up, you can remove a layer. Avoid anything that covers your neck, because when you flush it's harder for the heat to escape. Silk shirts or dresses aren't a good idea either, because any wet patches will be immediately visible.

24 Take control of the temperature

Make sure you stay cool at home and at the office by turning down the heating, turning on the air conditioning or opening a window.

Another useful item to have in your handbag is a hand-held, battery-operated fan. They're fairly cheap to buy and quickly cool you down.

25 Sleep tight

Hot flushes can disrupt your sleep. One minute you're too hot and removing your nightwear and casting aside your duvet, the next you're too cold and pulling everything back on! To minimise the risk of this happening, try the following simple actions:

- Keep your bedroom as cool as possible. Turn off the radiator. If your partner complains, point out that a cool room is conducive to sleep anyway.

- Use cotton bedding and nightwear. Sleep with a cotton sheet under your duvet. If a flush strikes, you can throw off the duvet and still be lightly covered.

- Keep a cool gel pack beneath your pillow at night – the type you can chill in the freezer. Turn your pillow over whenever you need to cool down.

- Keep a glass of cool water, perhaps with a sprig of refreshing mint, at your bedside and sip to replace fluids lost through night sweats. In really hot weather add ice and store in a thermos flask.

26 Don't be embarrassed

Finally, try not to feel embarrassed by a flush. Although you may feel unbearably hot and uncomfortable, it's likely that other people won't even notice.

To learn which foods and supplements may help to reduce flushing, see chapter 4. For alternative approaches to your menopausal symptoms, including flushing, see chapter 6.

Chapter 3

To HRT, or Not to HRT?

27 Consider whether to use HRT

HRT is a huge and highly controversial topic. The decision whether to take it or not is a personal one that only you can make. The arguments for and against HRT are complex. The better informed you are, the more likely you are to make the right choice for you. In this chapter, I've presented the key points. You'll find a basic explanation of what HRT is, a brief history, key study findings and criticisms, the potential risks and benefits and some experts' views. I've also suggested organisations you can consult for further information and opinions about HRT – the contact details are in the directory at the end of this book. You may want to read other books on the subject, so I've also listed some titles you may find helpful.

What is HRT?

HRT stands for Hormone Replacement Therapy. HRT comes in three main regimes – oestrogen only, cyclical combined and continuous combined – and in various forms, including pills, patches, pessaries, implants and gels.

Oestrogen-only HRT

This is usually prescribed for women who have had their womb removed (hysterectomy). HRT's beneficial effects come from oestrogen – progestogen is only added to protect the womb lining from the risk of cancer in women who still have their wombs intact. It is available in tablet, patch or gel form.

Cyclical combined HRT

This is where you take oestrogen each day and progestogen for 12 to 14 days of each cycle. It is normally offered if you are still having periods, or have had a period within the past year. This can be in oral, patch or gel form (with the addition of progestogen by tablet or a Mirena coil), or a combination of both, and leads to a bleed every 28 days. Long cycle HRT, also known as three-monthly HRT, involves taking oestrogen every day and progestogen for 12 to 14 days, every 13 weeks. This causes withdrawal bleeds every three months instead of every month, and is most suited to women who suffer side effects when taking progestogen. However, how safe it is in the long term is unclear.

Continuous combined HRT

If you haven't had a period for a year or longer, you'll probably be offered a continuous combined HRT, which means you take both oestrogen and progestogen each day. It's available as a pill, a patch or a gel (with the addition of progestogen by tablet or a Mirena coil). In theory, you shouldn't have a monthly bleed, but some women experience spotting, or mild and irregular bleeds for the first six months or so.

Benefits of using HRT patches/gels

HRT patches and gels are thought to be safer than tablets because the oestrogen is absorbed through the skin into the bloodstream, where it is diluted and broken down slowly before it reaches the liver, which reduces the risk of blood clots forming. These types of HRT are also better for women who suffer from migraines, as they keep hormone levels more stable than tablets and are therefore less likely to trigger attacks.

Local oestrogen

These include vaginal tablets, creams, pessaries or rings, which are used for treating uro-genital problems such as vaginal dryness, irritations or infections. Progestogen can also be used locally to protect the womb lining. Local oestrogen is thought to have a lower risk of side effects because it is less likely to be absorbed throughout the body; however its effects on the womb lining from long-term use are uncertain, so GPs are advised to pause the treatment at least once a year to review whether or not they still need to use it.

The oestrogen used in these preparations is chemically produced in a laboratory from pregnant mare's urine, soya or yams. Progestogen is a synthetic progesterone, often derived from plants such as yam, soya or sisal. Evidence suggests that the benefits of taking HRT include the prevention of hot flushes and night sweats, an improvement in hormonally related low mood, vaginal dryness and insomnia and a reduced risk of osteoporosis and bowel cancer.

Bioidentical hormones

Also known as individualised or bespoke HRT, the chemical structure of bioidentical hormones closely resembles that of the hormones your body would produce naturally. Proponents claim that they are therefore more natural than conventional HRT, so the body can metabolise them more easily, which means there are fewer side effects.

Bioidentical hormones can include oestrone, oestradiol, oestriol, testosterone, progesterone and other hormones such as dehydroepiandrosterone (DHEA), a hormone involved in the production of male and female sex hormones. They are dispensed as creams, capsules, drops applied to the tongue, and lozenges.

However, some experts point out that these hormones are made in a laboratory just like conventional HRT and from the same plant sources. The types and amounts of bioidentical hormones prescribed are calculated by measuring the hormone levels in each woman's saliva; critics argue that this is unlikely to give an accurate picture because hormone levels fluctuate in response to various factors including diet and time of day. Also salivary hormone levels may not accurately reflect those elsewhere in the body.

Another issue is that bioidentical hormones are not licensed in the UK so they can only be prescribed by private doctors. This means that, unlike conventional HRT, bioidentical hormones are currently not subjected to strict controls or regulations on their production, prescribing or dosage. Also, very little scientific information exists about their safety and effectiveness. In January 2008 the FDA (United States Food and Drug Administration) expressed concerns about the unsubstantiated claims made by manufacturers of bioidentical hormones regarding the safety, effectiveness and superiority of their products. In Australia several cases of womb cancer in women using bioidentical hormones have been reported. While some women report that this treatment works for them, it would seem that more research into its safety and effectiveness, and some form of regulation, are needed to ensure it is used safely.

Tibolone

Tibolone is a synthetic, tablet form of period-free HRT that mimics the actions of oestrogen and progesterone. Like continuous combined HRT, it is taken continuously and has similar effects. It has some androgenic (male hormone) effects too. It is also prescribed to help prevent osteoporosis. It is usually only prescribed for postmenopausal women for whom other forms of HRT are unsuitable.

A brief history of HRT

HRT originally consisted of oestrogen only and was first given by injection to alleviate menopausal symptoms in the 1930s. In 1942 an oral form was developed. For the next three decades HRT was a popular 'cure' for menopausal problems. In 1975 strong evidence of a link between oestrogen and womb cancer led to a decline in HRT use. Progestogen was added, with the aim of counteracting this effect and HRT was relaunched. Oestrogen alone is still offered to women who have had a hysterectomy. During the 1980s and early 1990s HRT regained popularity, amid reports that it prevented diseases such as osteoporosis and coronary heart disease.

By the late 1990s evidence of an increased risk of breast cancer and cardiovascular disease in the first year of use was emerging. Then the Women's Health Initiative (WHI) study in the US in 2002 and The Million Women Study in the UK in 2003, linked combined HRT use in 50- to 60-year-old women with a small increased risk of breast cancer, stroke, blood clots and coronary heart disease.

The Million Women Study later linked oestrogen-only HRT to a slightly increased risk of womb cancer and all types of HRT to an increased risk of ovarian cancer. Other studies reached similar conclusions. The WHI study also pointed to a reduction in bowel cancer and bone fractures among combined HRT users. Women who'd undergone a hysterectomy and were taking oestrogen-only HRT were not deemed to be at increased risk of breast cancer.

Between 2004 and 2007, the WHI published further analysis suggesting that some of the dangers had been over-estimated. A follow-up study in 2008 suggested a small increased risk in all cancers three years after stopping HRT treatment. The raised risk of a cardiovascular event seemed to disappear within three years of stopping HRT. The full study results also suggested that the increased risk for breast cancer was found only in those women who had taken HRT before taking part in the study.

Also, where the WHI study authors originally claimed there was no difference in effects according to age, further analyses from both the combined HRT and oestrogen-alone studies showed there was no increase in heart disease in women starting HRT within 10 years of the menopause.

A large controlled trial in Denmark backed up these findings, reporting that healthy women taking combined HRT for 10 years straight after the menopause had a lower risk of heart disease and of dying from it. The WHI study concluded that starting HRT after the age of 60 years may increase the risk of heart disease.

These studies suggest a 'window of opportunity' around the time of menopause when HRT should be started, as the health risks then are very small. However, the risks increase as women get older – so it is generally inadvisable for women over 60 to start HRT. But this doesn't mean that women who started taking HRT earlier should have to stop taking it when they reach 60.

Key study findings

The WHI study reported in 2002 that the additional yearly risks per 10,000 postmenopausal women taking combined HRT were: eight more cases of invasive breast cancer; seven more heart attacks; eight more strokes and eight more blood clots in the lung. The reduced risks (benefits) were: six fewer bowel cancers and five fewer hip fractures.

The Million Women Study, published in 2003, estimated that ten years' use of HRT resulted in five extra breast cancer cases per 1,000 oestrogen-only users and 19 more cancers per 1,000 users of combined oestrogen and progestogen.

Media hype

The significance of these studies can be hard to ascertain – especially when the media appear to sensationalise the findings. For example, in 2002 many newspapers reported that the risk of breast cancer in combined HRT users was 26 per cent higher than non-users. But this was the relative increased risk. In real terms it equated to an extra eight cases of breast cancer per 10,000 HRT users, per year.

Similarly, in 2008 the media reported that the risk of all cancers was 24 per cent higher three years after stopping HRT than among non-HRT users. In absolute terms, this equates to around three extra cases of any cancer per thousand combined HRT users each year. So the increased risks to health are small and this needs to be remembered when you're considering your options.

Study criticisms

It's not just the media's coverage of the studies' findings that's been criticised – the studies themselves have been deemed misleading.

One of the main criticisms of the WHI study has been that the average age of the participants was 63, which is over ten years older than the average menopausal woman embarking on HRT. Also, most of the women were overweight, with an average BMI of 28.5, which is a risk factor for heart disease and certain cancers, including breast cancer.

A re-evaluation of the WHI findings suggested that women aged 50 to 59 may not be at greater risk of heart disease.

The findings of the Million Women Study were challenged for focussing only on women who attended breast-screening appointments, which, it was suggested, increased the likelihood that it included a higher proportion of women with a family history of breast cancer.

Risks versus benefits

As with all medications, the overall risks versus the benefits need to be weighed up. In the case of HRT, the flaws in the research need to be taken into account too.

If you experience menopause before the age of 45, you have an increased risk of developing osteoporosis because in effect you've lost several years' worth of the bone-protective effects of oestrogen. HRT has been shown to reduce the risk of fractures, so in this case scenario the benefits could outweigh the risks. Also, some of the risks associated with HRT may be lower in this age group. In its Consensus Statement on HRT, The British Menopause Society Council remarks that an increase in breast cancer as a result of taking any type of HRT isn't seen among women who take HRT early, for premature menopause.

If, despite following a healthy lifestyle, your menopausal symptoms are so severe they're affecting your quality of life, the benefits of taking HRT may well outweigh the risks. HRT has been shown to prevent hot flushes and night sweats in most cases. It's also effective for relieving vaginal dryness and may help hormone-related depression and insomnia. Remember that the WHI study focussed on older women, so if you're in your 40s or 50s, the risks are likely to be lower. Also, The Million Women Study looked at the increased risk of breast cancer from ten years of HRT use – most women are now advised to take HRT for five years or less – and it may have included a high proportion of women with a familial link to breast cancer.

Possible side effects

Evidence suggests that possible side effects of taking combined HRT include bloating, breast tenderness, increased headaches/migraine – though some women report fewer – depression and some initial nausea. If you have fibroids they may increase in size. Rarely, equine oestrogens may raise blood pressure.

Such effects can be transient, so your GP may suggest you continue for a few months to see if the problems settle down. However, if you experience these effects persistently or suffer more serious ones, such as severe pain or breathlessness, see your GP or other medical professional as soon as possible.

Expert viewpoints

Menopause Matters, an independent website set up by gynaecologist and obstetrician Dr Heather Currie, aims to provide accurate information about the menopause and treatment options. The site, which contains contributions from clinicians who are experts in menopause management, provides a simple model of the risks and benefits of HRT and concludes: 'Generally though, if you become menopausal early (before age 45) or prematurely (before age 40), the benefits of taking HRT up to at least age 50 far outweigh the risks. If you are under 60 and having menopausal symptoms, the benefits also outweigh the risks.'

Marilyn Glenville, a leading nutritional therapist and exponent of natural alternatives to HRT, concedes in her book, *Natural Alternatives to HRT*, that women who have undergone a surgical menopause early in life may need HRT. She then argues that women going through a natural menopause, with or without a womb, are in a different position and asks, 'Are the benefits of HRT really worth the risk?' – before pointing out that there are lots of natural alternatives.

Janet Brockie, menopause nurse specialist at the John Radcliffe Hospital in Oxford, told me: 'I've always felt that women themselves need to take some responsibility for their own health, and sensible eating, lifestyle and exercise are vital. From meeting and talking to hundreds and probably thousands of women at this point in their lives, most women would prefer to avoid taking hormones, but some women do want them, need them and benefit from them. However, health professionals need to respect and embrace the wishes of those women that don't want or need HRT and hence it is important to consider alternatives.'

To help you weigh up the evidence, other organisations also offer expert opinions about the current research into HRT – these include The British Menopause Society, Women's Health Concern, Women's Health and The Natural Health Advisory Service. Contact details are in the directory at the end of this book.

Your choice

Whether you take HRT or not is your choice. The decision you make is likely to be influenced by factors such as how you view the menopause, the extent of your symptoms, how you feel about taking medication every day, and your perception of and attitude to the risks. If you feel strongly that HRT might help you, speak to your GP and discuss the pros and cons for you as an individual. Your GP should assess your personal risk of developing cancer or cardiovascular disease and take into account any other contraindications – for example suffering from migraines – before prescribing. Obviously, you should only take HRT for as long as you need to. The current recommendation is that women should use the lowest effective dose for the shortest possible time – usually less than five years – though some women may need to take it for longer. Women using HRT should also have annual reviews with their GP to assess the treatment's effectiveness and whether they are suffering any adverse effects.

You may opt for HRT and then, perhaps as a result of side effects, decide it's not for you. Or you may find you can't do without it – like the actress Jane Seymour. Jane took HRT from the age of 47 to tackle her hot flushes and irritability. In 2005, after seven years, she stopped taking it, amid fears over its safety. Despite following a healthy lifestyle, her symptoms returned within months. In the end, she weighed up the pros and cons and opted for a lower dose of HRT, via a patch, and a diet rich in phytoestrogens to control her symptoms. She concluded, 'Everyone was telling me different things, but I realised that each woman has to create her own way of dealing with the menopause, one that she is comfortable with.'

Chapter 4

Natural HRT

Whether you opt for HRT or not, evidence suggests that tailoring your diet and lifestyle can help to control the symptoms of the menopause. We've already looked at how a poor diet can exacerbate, or even cause, hot flushes. An inadequate diet may also contribute to other menopausal symptoms and common postmenopausal diseases, such as cardiovascular disease, breast cancer and osteoporosis. This chapter looks at foods you can eat and supplements you can take that may help to prevent, or alleviate, many of these problems and provide an alternative to HRT, or complement it.

Stay hydrated

Drinking enough water is always important, whatever your age, but ensuring you drink enough before, during and after the menopause can help to prevent the development of other conditions that can be a problem at this time, such as cystitis and migraine. Your brain is 80 per cent water, so drinking enough helps ensure its healthy function. It's especially important to replace the fluid lost through flushing and night sweats. The Food Standards Agency recommends that we drink at least 1.2 litres of fluid per day.

28 Balance your hormones with phytoestrogens

Phytoestrogens are plant oestrogens that appear to have an oestrogenic or anti-oestrogenic effect. Bacteria in the gut convert these plant hormones into substances that may provide similar benefits to oestrogen. The three main types of phytoestrogens are isoflavones, lignans and coumestans. The four most active isoflavones appear to be genistein, daidzein, biochanin A and formononetin. The best sources of isoflavones are pulses. Lignans are obtained mainly from cereals, fruit, vegetables and seeds. Coumestans are largely found in bean sprouts and are less common in British and American diets.

Women in parts of Asia who eat lots of foods containing these phytonutrients, such as soya, rice and vegetables, seem to have fewer menopausal symptoms. The breast cancer rate is also much lower – about a quarter of that occurring in the UK and US. Research suggests that women in the UK and US have an average daily isoflavone intake of 4.5 mg, whereas the average Japanese woman's intake each day is 50 mg, and in some cases can be as high as 100 mg.

There's evidence to suggest that some, but not all, women benefit from eating more of these foods, or taking phytoestrogen rich supplements, with up to 40 per cent fewer hot flushes, stronger bones and softer skin. A review of 13 studies concluded that women who suffer from frequent flushes benefit the most. It seems some women absorb phytoestrogens better than others. Not smoking and drinking alcohol in moderation helps. Antibiotics can hinder absorption, because they destroy beneficial bacteria. Eating foods that provide prebiotics (e.g. tomatoes) and probiotics (e.g. bio-yogurt) can increase absorption, especially after a course of antibiotics. Also, eating less fat and more carbohydrates seems beneficial. Studies show that eating such a diet increases the conversion of daidzein into equol, a substance with oestrogenic effects.

Beneficial bugs

Prebiotics contain carbohydrates, which feed and encourage the growth of 'good' bacteria in the gut. They're found in everyday foods such as onions, tomatoes, leeks, garlic, cucumber, celery, bananas and oats. These foods also contain phytoestrogens. Probiotics, such as *Lactobacillus* or *Streptococcus*, are now added to many foods and drinks, but these can be expensive – eating natural, live bio-yogurt is a cheap and easy way of including them in your diet.

Super soya

Soya is a particularly rich source of two types of isoflavones – genistein and daidzein. Eating soya products may benefit your health both before and after the menopause. A study showed that women who ate 45 g of soya daily had 40 per cent fewer hot flushes. Soya beans contain all eight amino acids, making them a complete protein. They're also rich in essential fatty acids. They've been shown to reduce cholesterol, thus protecting against heart disease, and may lower the risk of hormone-related cancers such as breast cancer.

You can include soya in your diet quite easily. Try replacing cow's milk with soya milk – most are fortified with calcium, which provides added protection against osteoporosis. You could also try soya-based yogurts, cheeses and desserts. Tofu is soya bean curd, made from coagulated soya milk. It's bland taste makes it versatile, but it needs to be accompanied by strong tasting ingredients to give it flavour. There are two types – one is firm and dense and can be used in stir-fries, soups and salads. The other – silken tofu – has a softer texture and can be used for spreads, dips, sauces, desserts and smoothies.

Substitute soya mince for meat when cooking. The recommended daily amount of isoflavones is 45 mg – 55 g of tofu or 600 ml of soya milk yields around 40 mg. A 100 g portion of soya beans contains about 37 mg of isoflavones. Try them in casseroles, stews and salads. Dried soya beans need to be soaked overnight. Tinned ones can be used, but if they have added salt rinse them first. Miso, a paste made from fermented soya beans that can be used like a stock cube to add flavour to stews, soups and casseroles, is a concentrated source of isoflavones. Soy sauce, also produced from fermented soya beans, contributes small amounts of isoflavones when added to dishes like stir-fries or noodles. It should only be used sparingly, however, as it is high in salt. Soya flakes have a nutty flavour – try sprinkling them over cereal, or add them to home-made muesli.

A soya milk fruit smoothie is a great way to include both phytoestrogens and more fruit in your diet. Because you're blending, rather than juicing, you get the benefits of the whole fruit, including the fibre. You can add any fruit you like – apricots, strawberries, peaches, pears and cherries taste good in a smoothie and are rich in phytoestrogens. Cinnamon not only adds flavour, but boosts the phytoestrogen content too – see the Recipes section.

If you dislike soya products, or find that diet alone doesn't improve your symptoms, consider taking a supplement with soya isoflavones and other phytoestrogens.

Eat out Japanese style

Eat at a Japanese restaurant and you can feast on foods that will help you beat many menopausal symptoms. Choose miso soup, edamame (fresh soya beans in the pod) and tofu to combat flushes, and sushi and sashimi to boost your intake of oily fish and help protect against depression and heart disease.

Chickpea chick

Chickpeas contain all four types of isoflavones, so they're well worth including in your diet. Use them to add interest to stews, curries, pastas and salads, or use them instead of rice to stuff peppers or tomatoes. Hummus contains chickpeas and makes a great dip, or sandwich filler. You can buy it in most supermarkets, or you can make your own – see the Recipes section.

Full of beans

As well as soya, all kinds of beans are good sources of isoflavones and also supply smaller amounts of lignans and coumestans. You don't need to eat the more exotic aduki and mung beans – the ever popular baked bean, haricot beans, butter beans and kidney beans appear to be just as beneficial. See the Recipes section for a mixed bean salad recipe.

Let's have lentils

Lentils contain all four classes of isoflavones as well as some lignans and coumestans. They're also high in fibre. There are various types, including red, green, brown, orange and black. Try adding them to curries, soups and broths. Unlike other dried pulses, they don't need soaking first. The warm lentil salad in the Recipes section contains olive oil and tomatoes, which also provide lignans.

Peas please

Like lentils, peas contain isoflavones and fibre, so they're worth eating regularly. If you're bored with serving them as a side vegetable, you can add them to lots of dishes including risottos, kedgeree, omelettes, pizzas, pastas, soups, salads, casseroles and curries.

Our daily bread

A recent study showed that bread is one of the main sources of isoflavones in women's diets in the UK. Whilst bread doesn't contain massive amounts of these phytonutrients, it makes a useful contribution to our daily intake. This may be due in part to the widespread addition of soya flour to bread in the UK. Wholemeal bread provides the most genistein and daidzein and, as it's an unrefined cereal, also supplies lignans. Lignan levels are highest in unrefined grains. Yet more reasons to eat wholemeal, rather than white bread! Multigrain breads, such as Burgen soya and linseed, and rye breads, are also good sources of phytoestrogens.

Rice is nice

Wholegrain brown rice is a good source of genistein and daidzein and contains some lignans too. Try serving it instead of white rice with stir-fries, chilli and curries. It has a delicious nutty flavour, but if you find the taste difficult to adjust to try mixing it with an equal amount of white rice at first and gradually reduce the quantity. For best results, soak brown rice in water for about 25 minutes before cooking. This softens the outer bran layer so that it cooks more quickly.

Veg out

Eating a variety of vegetables is not just good for your general health – it can also reduce menopausal symptoms.

Brassicas (cabbage, broccoli, cauliflower, kale and Brussels sprouts) are good sources of lignans. French beans, carrots, green and red peppers and courgettes also provide decent amounts. Cucumber and tomatoes provide some – but tomato paste is a more concentrated source. Eating vegetables raw or stir-fried provides the most lignans, whilst boiling lowers the amount.

Some vegetables (e.g. broccoli and tomatoes) also contain the isoflavones genistein and daidzein. Cabbage contains another less common class of phytoestrogens called coumarins.

Green vegetables also contain glucosinolates, which may protect against breast cancer. One portion contains the recommended daily amount. For optimum glucosinolate content, use fresh vegetables that have been stored in the fridge and steam, stir-fry, or microwave, rather than boiling.

Drink tomato juice

In 2015 a study at Tokyo Medical University involving 93 women showed that drinking 200 ml of tomato juice twice daily for eight weeks almost halved their menopausal symptoms, including anxiety, hot flushes and irritability, and lowered their cholesterol levels. It's thought tomato juice not only provides plant oestrogens, but also gamma-aminobutyric acid (GABA), which has a calming effect on the brain.

Be fruitful

Eat fruit, not only for the usual associated benefits, such as vitamins and fibre, but also for their phytoestrogen content. Apricots, strawberries, blackberries, cranberries, peaches, pears, nectarines, pink grapefruit, cherries, kiwis and plums are especially high in lignans, though most other fruits contain some.

A sprinkling of seeds

Sprinkle one or two tablespoons of linseeds, otherwise known as flaxseeds, over cereals, salads, yogurt or even stir-fries to relieve menopausal symptoms. Nutty flavoured linseeds are the best source of lignans and contain omega-3 oils and fibre, so they could help relieve hot flushes as well as protect against heart disease and help maintain gut and general health. Burgen soya and linseed bread is a good way of gaining the benefits of both soya and linseed in one go and is a good source of calcium and fibre. Other seeds, especially sesame and sunflower, are also good sources of lignans. Raw seeds contain the most – baking or roasting them seems to reduce the lignan content. But if you find raw linseeds difficult to chew, you can buy them roasted and still benefit from decent amounts of lignans.

Oat so good

Another way of increasing your phytoestrogen intake is to include oats in your diet. Oats are a good source of lignans. They also contain soluble fibre, which lowers blood cholesterol and is less likely to irritate the gut if you suffer from irritable bowel syndrome (IBS).

Note

Some women find their IBS worsens, or they suffer from the condition for the first time during the menopause. This is because the muscles in the gut have oestrogen receptors and can therefore lose tone as oestrogen levels fall, leading to digestive problems such as diarrhoea or constipation, nausea and indigestion.

Porridge makes a satisfying breakfast, or try an oat-based granola type cereal. You can also buy oatcakes, which make a healthy snack. The soluble fibre in oats is also a prebiotic, so it encourages the growth of immunity boosting 'good' bacteria which also help ease IBS symptoms.

Go for garlic

Garlic is a good source of lignans. It can be used to add flavour to many dishes: pastas, stir-fries and pizzas, to name but a few. Garlic also contains sulphur compounds, including allicin, which are believed to protect against cardiovascular disease by lowering cholesterol and may lower the risk of stomach and bowel cancers.

Opt for olive oil

Olive oil features heavily in Mediterranean diets, which have been linked to longevity and a reduced risk of cancers and cardiovascular disease. This may be at least partly due to the lignans it contains. Extra virgin olive oil provides the most. Enjoy its sweet, spicy flavour in salad dressings and stir-fries, or use it as a dip with crusty wholemeal bread.

Safe frying

There has recently been a lot of debate regarding which oils are the healthiest for cooking with. This is because when oils are heated to high temperatures they produce toxic substances called aldehydes, which are linked to cancer, heart disease and dementia. The most recent research, conducted in 2015 at De Montfort University in Leicester for the BBC programme *Trust Me, I'm A Doctor*, suggests that olive, rapeseed and coconut oils produce the least aldehydes at high temperatures, while corn and sunflower oils form the most. Always store oils in a cupboard away from light, and avoid reusing oils, to prevent the formation of aldehydes.

Taste of the orient

The common or garden bean sprouts – germinated mung beans – often used in Asian cooking are rich in coumestans and isoflavones. They're best eaten as soon as possible after purchase, as they lose their crispness fairly quickly. Add them to sandwiches and salads for extra crunch, or try the tofu, vegetable and bean sprout stir fry in the recipes section for a quick, phytoestrogen rich meal.

Caribbean cuisine

Yams may help to promote hormonal balance. They contain diosgenin, which is used in laboratories to produce progestogen – a synthetic version of progesterone. Whilst the body can't make progesterone from diosgenin, it's thought to have a balancing effect on progesterone and oestrogen levels. Yams are a staple food in the Caribbean. They taste similar to sweet potatoes and can be served like potatoes – mashed, baked or as chips baked in the oven with olive oil.

Beneficial tipple

The polyphenols in red wine are thought to protect against atherosclerosis (hardening of the arteries), which can lead to cardiovascular disease. Research also suggests that red wine may reduce the risk of stomach cancer and Alzheimer's. But women going through the menopause have yet another excuse for enjoying a regular glass of red – it's a decent source of lignans as well. Remember that moderation is key – more than three units daily or fourteen units weekly may increase your risk of breast cancer and cardiovascular disease and have other ill effects; alcohol can also disrupt sleep, affecting the chemical messengers that appear to influence sleep. One small (125 ml) glass of wine contains on average 1.5 units of alcohol. A large glass (175 ml) typically contains two units. A 250 ml glass contains about three units.

Tea time

If you enjoy a cuppa, you'll be pleased to know that tea is a decent source of lignans, as well as antioxidants. Black teas contain more than green tea. This may partly explain why some studies have shown that drinking tea helps to protect against osteoporosis. Coffee also contains lignans, but in lower concentrations. There's evidence that black and green tea can help prevent Alzheimer's too.

Drinking more than six cups of tea or three to four cups of coffee a day may have a negative effect on your bones due to the caffeine content – see tip 32. Find out how to keep your bones healthy further on in this chapter.

Sprinkle cinnamon

Sprinkle cinnamon on desserts and hot and cold drinks to benefit from the plant oestrogens it contains. It's also thought to thin the blood and reduce cholesterol, thus lowering the risk of heart attacks and stroke. It could help to keep the blood sugar steady and may even ease joint stiffness and pain.

29 Eat foods that lift your mood

Declining oestrogen and progesterone levels are thought to contribute to low mood. To help avoid depression and anxiety it's important to eat foods that provide the nutrients essential to healthy brain function.

- Oily fish, such as sardines, salmon and mackerel, and nuts, seeds and vegetable oils contain essential fatty acids, which are vital for healthy brain function. Avoid low-fat diets – research suggests that drastically reducing all types of fat in the diet can cause anxiety and depression.

- Foods with a low glycaemic index (GI), such as oats and wholewheat cereals, bread and pasta, help maintain a steady blood sugar and avoid the irritability and depression that can result from low blood sugar. These carbohydrates also help the body make serotonin, a brain chemical that boosts mood and self-esteem.

- Bananas, avocados, chicken and turkey are rich in tryptophan and vitamin B6, which the body uses to make mood-enhancing serotonin. Eggs, beans, lentils, nuts and seeds also contain tryptophan.

- Dairy foods are rich in calcium, which induces calm, as well as tryptophan, making them a great mood booster.

- B vitamins ensure a healthy nervous system and stave off depression. Wholegrains, meat, fish, dairy foods, nuts, seeds, beans and green vegetables and citrus fruits will provide all the B vitamins.

- Nuts, wholegrains, beans and green leafy vegetables are rich in magnesium. A lack of magnesium can lead to anxiety and depression.

- Include selenium-rich foods such as Brazil nuts, shellfish and liver. A low selenium intake has been linked to depression.

- Basil is widely used by herbalists as an anti-depressant. Add torn basil leaves to pastas, pizzas and salads.

- Chocolate increases serotonin (a mood and sleep-enhancing substance) in the brain. Plain chocolate is the healthiest, as milk chocolate contains fewer flavanols and more fat and sugar.

- Vanilla also has a calming effect. Try drinking hot milk with pure vanilla extract.

- *Melissa officinalis*, commonly known as lemon balm because of its nettle-like, lemon-scented leaves, has soothing and calming properties which help to ease tension, anxiety and headaches and enhance mood. It's also believed to boost memory by making brain cells more receptive to acetylcholine, a brain chemical linked to memory. The leaves can be finely chopped and added to meat or fish dishes, or drunk hot or cold as a refreshing tea. Try blending them into a melon or pear smoothie to enhance the flavour.

30 Boost your memory

Studies involving soya-based foods suggest that the phyto-estrogens which they contain can improve memory at menopause. It's believed that this is because oestrogen is involved in memory function and plant hormones can fulfil a similar role. A number of other foods may also boost your brain power.

Power up with protein

Protein foods such as fish, lean meat, eggs, beans and nuts help your brain to stay alert and focussed. This is because they contain amino acids, which promote the release of neurotransmitters, whose job it is to transmit information within the brain and to other parts of the body. Aim at two to three servings of protein daily – preferably during the day, to help your brain function at its best. Eggs also contain phospholipids – fats which boost memory.

Berry good

The vitamins and anthocyanins in berries such as blueberries, raspberries and strawberries appear to prevent age-related brain deterioration and may improve short-term memory and restore coordination. Berries also contain phytoestrogens.

You should cocoa

Studies show that good-quality dark chocolate contains flavanols, which appear to boost blood flow to the brain, improving brain function and counteracting fatigue. For maximum health benefits go for chocolate containing 70 per cent or more cocoa. As an added benefit, plain chocolate is a decent source of lignans. To manage your weight, aim at eating no more than 25 g daily, as even dark chocolate can be high in fat and sugar.

Folic acid

Folic acid, otherwise known as folate, has been shown to slow down mental decline. The best sources include beetroot, broccoli, green vegetables, nuts and cereals.

Beneficial Brazils

Brazil nuts are a particularly good source of selenium, believed to protect against Alzheimer's, as well as depression and cancer. Like other nuts, they're packed with essential vitamins and minerals.

Favour curry

Turmeric, otherwise known as curcumin, is a member of the ginger family and a basic ingredient in curry. Research indicates that turmeric protects the brain from oxidation damage, protecting against memory loss and possibly Alzheimer's. Try adding turmeric powder to natural yogurt to use as a dressing with raw vegetables. Use it in stir-fries and home-made, low-fat curries.

31 Reduce symptoms with vitamin E and unsaturated fats

As well as phytoestrogens, foods containing vitamin E and unsaturated fats may help to reduce hot flushes and other symptoms.

Eat nuts and seeds for vitamin E

One study suggests that vitamin E may reduce flushing slightly. It may also help vaginal dryness. Vitamin E may also help prevent cataracts, Alzheimer's and heart disease. Just 15 hazel nuts provide the recommended daily intake of vitamin E for women. Pumpkin and sunflower seeds also provide phytoestrogens, protein, essential fatty acids, vitamins B and E and minerals, especially magnesium, making them an ideal snack during the menopause. Seeded breads or crisp breads, like Warburtons Seeded Batch Loaf and Ryvita Pumpkin Seeds and Oats, provide a convenient way to include them in your diet. Vitamin E oil can also relieve vagina dryness when applied to the area. If you use capsules, check they're yeast free to avoid yeast infections.

Nuts and seeds are quite high in calories, so try not to exceed one handful of nuts (around 300 calories) or two tablespoons of seeds (around 200 calories) daily. If you prefer, you can take a supplement of up to 1000 iu (international units) of natural vitamin E daily.

Avocado advantage

Avocados are also rich in vitamin E. They're high in monounsaturated fat, which lowers bad (LDL) cholesterol and raises good (HDL) cholesterol. This means they're quite high in calories, so restrict your portion size to half an avocado. They also contain the antioxidant beta-carotene, B vitamins, including folate, vitamin C and iodine, for healthy thyroid function. Try them added to salads, or make an avocado dip – see the Recipes section.

Avoid 'bad' fats

Avoid the saturated fats found in processed meats – especially sausages, bacon and burgers – as these are linked with coronary heart disease and stroke, atherosclerosis and certain cancers, including breast cancer. However, recent research suggests that some of the saturated fats found in full-fat dairy products such as whole milk, butter and yogurt and grass-fed, free range meat sources such as lamb, beef and wild game such as duck and venison may boost health; they are thought to cut the risk of diabetes and heart disease and help weight management by keeping you fuller for longer. Butter (especially grass-fed) is also a good source of vitamin A. Trans-fats, also known as partially hydrogenated fats, are also best avoided. These are formed when liquid vegetable oils are turned into solid fats, through a process known as hydrogenation and are linked to weight gain around the middle, hardened arteries, heart disease, diabetes and certain cancers.

Go for 'good' fats

Include 'good' unsaturated fats in your diet. Unsaturated fats appear to protect against many of the problems associated with the menopause and beyond, including hot flushes, dry skin, heart disease, stroke, osteoporosis, aches and pains and Alzheimer's.

There are two sorts of unsaturated fat: polyunsaturated essential fatty acids – omega-3 and omega-6 – and mono-unsaturated fat – omega-9. Omega-3 fats are thought to boost brain function by improving blood flow to the brain, and to reduce the risk of heart disease by lowering triglyceride levels. Research suggests they also strengthen the bones and are anti-inflammatory, reducing general aches and pains and those associated with arthritis and headaches. Oily fish, nuts, seeds, egg yolks, dark green leafy vegetables, hemp seed oil and linseed oil are good sources. Aim at eating these foods regularly, but if for some reason you can't manage to do this, it might be worth considering taking cod liver oil capsules.

Note: cod liver oil also contains vitamins A and D, so don't take it with other supplements containing these vitamins, as they're fat soluble. This means any excess is stored in the liver. Too much of these vitamins can be harmful.

Omega-6 fats are thought to help relieve menopausal symptoms by promoting hormonal balance. They're found in oils, such as evening primrose, linseed, sunflower and corn, nuts, olives, seeds and some grains.

Monounsaturated fats, also known as omega-9 fats, reduce LDL cholesterol, which is linked to heart disease and stroke. Good sources of omega-9 fats include olives and olive, rapeseed and peanut oils, avocados, nuts and seeds.

32 Keep your bones healthy

Oestrogen promotes bone renewal and improves calcium absorption into the bones, so the reduced levels associated with the menopause mean you're more at risk of osteoporosis. The phytoestrogen rich foods already mentioned could have similar effects on the bones as oestrogen, so eating these foods may benefit your bones, as well as your menopausal symptoms. To help slow bone loss after the menopause you also need to ensure an adequate intake of calcium, vitamin D, magnesium and zinc. Let's now look at the foods that provide these nutrients.

Bone builders

Calcium strengthens the bones. It's recommended that postmenopausal women have around 1,500 mg of calcium daily. The richest sources of calcium are dairy foods – especially low-fat milk, low-fat hard cheese and yogurt. Tinned sardines are a good source – if you eat the bones. Good non-animal calcium providers include almonds, seeds, tofu, soya, seaweed, figs, dates, dried apricots, Brazil nuts, purple broccoli, watercress, leeks, parsnips, lentils and beans and green leafy vegetables such as kale.

Vitamin D is essential for calcium absorption. It's produced by the body, following exposure to sunlight. Margarines, cereals and powdered milk are generally fortified with vitamin D. Other sources include liver and oily fish. The recommended daily allowance is between 400 and 800 iu.

Magnesium is involved in converting vitamin D to the active form needed to ensure calcium absorption, thus helping maintain bone density. Nuts, wholegrains and leafy green vegetables are good sources. Around 60 per cent of the magnesium in your body is stored in your bones.

Zinc stimulates bone formation. Meat, wholegrains, dairy foods, nuts and seeds are good sources.

Sprinkle leafy green vegetables with a little ordinary vinegar to increase your absorption of the calcium they contain. Drinking a tablespoon of cider vinegar and honey in warm water once or twice a day is also recommended for increasing calcium absorption. 'Good' bacteria – probiotics such as *Lactobacillus* – seem to improve calcium absorption. There are lots of probiotic foods and drinks on the market, but they can be expensive – natural live bio-yogurt is a good, relatively cheap source. Eating prebiotic foods such as onions, tomatoes, leeks, garlic, cucumber, celery and bananas, which feed and encourage the growth of probiotics in the gut, could also help. Don't forget, calcium is found in water – especially in hard water areas and some bottled waters.

Note: it's recommended that your daily calcium intake doesn't exceed more than 2,000 to 2,500 mg. A higher intake may interfere with the absorption of other minerals, such as iron, and could lead to other problems.

Don't overdo protein

Many nutritionists argue that eating too many protein foods can increase your risk of osteoporosis. This is because protein foods form acids which your body neutralises with alkaline minerals, including calcium from your bones. The more protein you eat, the more calcium you need. Salt is also thought to leach calcium from your bones. So don't overdo protein foods, or salt. Eat plenty of alkaline foods, for example fruit and vegetables, natural yogurt, brazil nuts, seeds and almonds.

Drink alcohol in moderation

Moderate drinking can boost blood oestrogen levels and improve bone strength. But drinking more than the recommended 14 units of alcohol per week can deplete calcium in the bones, reduce calcium absorption and reduce bone formation.

Avoid too much coffee

Drinking more than three to four cups of coffee daily could have a negative impact on your bone health. Studies suggest that a daily intake of 300 mg of caffeine can lead to loss of calcium, and magnesium in the urine. The average cup of instant or percolated coffee contains around 75 mg of caffeine. A mug contains around 100 mg – an espresso could have as much as 150 mg.

Forget the fizz

Avoid fizzy drinks, such as cola and lemonade, as they contain phosphates, which appear to block the absorption of calcium and may also trigger the release of calcium from the bones. Try to drink plain water instead.

Calcium supplements

It's always best to try to obtain essential vitamins and minerals from your diet, but if you're concerned that you don't eat enough calcium-rich foods, consider taking a calcium supplement. Avoid supplements containing calcium carbonate, as they can increase your chances of developing kidney stones. Opt instead for those containing calcium citrate, which is more easily absorbed, such as Solgar Calcium Citrate with Vitamin D.

Note: don't exceed 2,500 mg, as it could increase your risk of developing kidney stones and interfere with your absorption of minerals such as iron.

Other risk factors

Osteoporosis has been dubbed 'the silent disease' because most people with the condition aren't aware they have it. So being aware of the risk factors is important. The impact of the menopause and diet on the bones has already been covered – other risk factors for osteoporosis include:

- Being female (it affects one in three women).

- Early, or premature menopause.

- Being small boned, or underweight.

- A sedentary lifestyle.

- A family history of osteoporosis.

- Being over 65.

- Some medications, such as corticosteroids, anti-epileptic drugs and tranquilisers, may increase your risk.

Bone check

If you're concerned that you may be at risk, or if you break a bone after the menopause, it's advisable to ask your GP if you can have a DEXA (Dual Energy X-ray Absorptiometry) scan to check your bone density. An obvious sign of bone loss is a decrease in your height.

Further information is available from The National Osteoporosis Society, or Osteoporosis Advice – details are at the end of the book.

Salt warning

A high intake of salt is linked with high blood pressure, which increases your risk of coronary heart disease and stroke. Excess salt may also lead to osteoporosis, as well as stomach cancer and ulcers, and kidney problems. It's recommended we eat no more than 6 g of salt daily, but this can be difficult to achieve if you eat a lot of processed and pre-packaged foods. Sausages, bacon and hard cheeses are examples of salty foods. Some breakfast cereals can be worryingly high in salt. Many pre-packed sandwiches contain between 2.5 g and 4 g of salt. Some 400 g cans of soup contain 4 g. Regular-sized tins of baked beans (400 g) often contain 5 g of salt. The best way to cut your salt intake is to eat meals prepared and cooked at home, using little or no salt. Try using herbs, such as basil and rosemary, and spices such as garlic, ginger and chilli to add flavour to your cooking. Lime and lemon juice taste good when added to stir-fries and fish dishes. Foods which are canned in brine should always be rinsed and then heated through in water before consumption.

Check labels

If you must eat processed foods and ready meals, check the labels and choose those with no more than 0.3 g of salt per 100 g. There are lower salt versions of many foods including soups, baked beans and tomato ketchup.

Note: many food manufacturers list the sodium content, which must be multiplied by 2.5 to work out the salt content. Often the sodium or salt content per 100 g is given, which again involves maths to work out the total amount in the product.

Aka salt

Salt comes under many guises. Products with any of these ingredients may be high in salt: monosodium glutamate; disodium phosphate; brine; garlic salt; onion salt; sodium benzoate; sodium alginate; sodium hydroxide; sodium caseinate; sodium nitrate; sodium pectinate; sodium propionate; sodium sulphite; soy sauce; baking powder; baking soda.

33 Eat to ease cystitis

Many women suffer from cystitis more often both during the perimenopause and postmenopause. Declining oestrogen levels lead to thinning of the urethra and vagina linings and less mucous in the vagina, both of which make infections more likely.

Cystitis is usually due to a bacterial infection causing inflammation in the lining of the bladder and urethra. The symptoms include wanting to urinate more often – even when the bladder is empty, a burning and stinging feeling when passing urine, lower abdominal pain and dark, cloudy, or strong-smelling urine. In severe cases there can be blood in the urine, fever and a feeling of unwellness.

Various foods and drinks are thought to be helpful in the prevention and treatment of cystitis:

- Garlic has an antibiotic effect, helping to control cystitis-causing bacteria such as *E. coli* and *Staphylococcus*.

- Natural bio-yogurt containing *Lactobacillus acidophilus* is helpful. It introduces beneficial bacteria to the gut, boosting immunity and helping the body to resist infection. It may also help promote a healthy balance of good bacteria in the bladder. When applied to the vagina it's thought to help restore the natural pH balance.

- Watermelon and celery have a gentle diuretic effect, which can help flush the bacteria from the bladder.

- Drinking cranberry juice can help both prevent and treat cystitis. Cranberries contain anthocyanins, powerful antioxidants with antibacterial properties. Tannins in cranberries discourage bacteria from sticking to the mucous membranes of the bladder and urethra and multiplying, helping to prevent urinary tract infections.

- Try drinking a tumbler of water with one teaspoon of bicarbonate of soda dissolved in it three times daily, until the symptoms subside. It works by making your urine less acidic, which reduces the burning sensation and inhibits harmful bacterial growth.

- A tea made by pouring boiling water over two teaspoons of fresh thyme, which is antibacterial, is also recommended.

- Avoid drinking too much tea, coffee and alcohol, as these can irritate the bladder.

If symptoms persist, or you notice blood in your urine, see your GP. For practical tips on preventing and treating cystitis, see 'Stop cystitis' in chapter 5.

The menopause diet

To sum up, a healthy, balanced diet containing fruit, vegetables, pulses, wholegrains, nuts and seeds, with small amounts of dairy foods, eggs, oily fish, lean meats and unsaturated oils and little salt, sugar and trans-fats, will help to reduce menopausal symptoms and ensure a healthy old age. There's no need for deprivation – you can indulge in a glass of red wine, a cup of tea, or a little plain chocolate, knowing that they contain beneficial compounds.

If you're on a restricted budget, focus on cheap but nutritious ingredients such as pulses, potatoes, brown rice, oats, wholemeal bread and pasta. Eggs, baked beans, tinned sardines and tuna are low-cost sources of protein and other nutrients. These foods can form the basis of family meals – such as stir-fries, broths, casseroles and pasta dishes – and will help prevent weight gain and ensure you look your best. See chapter 7 to learn how the foods you eat can benefit your appearance.

34 Seek help from herbs

Various herbs, many of which contain phytoestrogens, have traditionally been used to reduce menopausal symptoms. However, in some cases the evidence is only anecdotal. Some women benefit from taking phytoestrogens, others – about 50 per cent – don't, because they can't metabolise it in the gut. It's important to remember that just because something is natural, it doesn't necessarily mean it's safe – many plants are poisonous to humans. Herbal remedies are medicines, and like any medicine, may have adverse effects. They may also interact with other medications. Always inform your GP if you are taking herbal medicines.

Janet Brockie, menopause nurse specialist at the John Radcliffe Hospital in Oxford, says: 'The big issue is the effectiveness of alternatives and potential for harm. This includes side effects, but also doing harm because an alternative treatment chosen, instead of a known effective orthodox treatment, fails to be effective – an example of this is a woman at risk of osteoporosis thinking she is protecting her bones by eating soy or another woman thinking that progesterone cream will protect the lining of her womb, while she is also taking oestrogen.'

She adds, 'We should be cautious about unsupported claims about alternatives; however, sometimes there is no evidence because the research just hasn't been done. So when there is no evidence about an alternative treatment, it doesn't automatically mean that something isn't safe or effective – we often just simply do not know, but need to bear in mind it might be harmful. Sadly, there are not the resources or infrastructure for research into alternative medicine in the same way as in orthodox medicine.'

Are supplements safe?

Herbal products are generally sold as either traditional herbal registration (THR) remedies or herbal food supplements. THR products are regulated and monitored by the government agency known as the Medicines and Healthcare products Regulatory Authority. If a product has a THR stamp it means the MHRA is satisfied it meets quality standards, has appropriate labelling and a product information leaflet. It also indicates that the herb has been used in traditional remedies for over 30 years. All THR products have a nine-digit registration number starting with the letters THR on the container or packaging.

Herbal food supplements come under the remit of the Food Standards Agency (FSA) and the Chartered Trading Standards Institute at local authority level and are not under the same legal and manufacturing scrutiny. This means there is no guarantee of their content or quality. In 2015 the School of Pharmacy at University College London tested over 70 of the herbal remedies most often bought from the high street or online and found that while most contained high amounts of the main ingredient, worryingly up to a third had very little or none at all. So it is probably best to choose THR remedies or, if a product isn't registered, check that it is from a reputable company.

Also, a few herbal medicines in the UK have a product licence. Licensed herbal medicines, like any other medicine, are required to demonstrate safety, quality and effectiveness, and to provide guidelines on safe use; only herbal medicines with medicinal claims supported by acceptable clinical data are given product licences. They can be identified by a nine-digit number, prefixed by the letters PL.

There is a full list of herbal medicines granted a traditional herbal registration on the MHRA website, as well as further advice and information about using herbal medicines safely. The contact details are in the directory at the end of this book.

Check the benefits

To determine whether it is worth carrying on taking a herbal medicine or supplement, check the effects it has on your menopausal symptoms. Rate each of your symptoms from zero to ten before you start taking the herbal medicine/supplement and then repeat after three months to see if your symptoms have improved – if they haven't, stop taking it.

Agnus castus

Agnus castus is derived from the berries of the chaste tree, a shrub native to West Asia and south-western Europe, which was introduced to English gardens in the sixteenth century. It has long been used to relieve PMT and menopausal symptoms. It's claimed to balance female hormones by stimulating the pituitary gland, which produces and sets hormone level, helping to combat flushes and night sweats. However, there doesn't seem to be any clear evidence regarding the benefits of its use.

Black cohosh

Black cohosh is a member of the buttercup family that grows in North America, where it's widely used by native Americans to treat gynaecological problems. It's believed to have oestrogenic properties and to be particularly effective for the treatment of hot flushes and depression.

Several studies suggest that black cohosh can reduce hot flushes and night sweats. Some link its effects to its oestrogenic actions, others to its ability to lower luteinising hormone levels, which rise at menopause. One US study suggests it influences body temperature by targeting serotonin receptors. In Germany, the Commission E, an expert committee set up to evaluate the safety and effectiveness of herbal remedies, recommends taking black cohosh for menopausal symptoms for six months.

The evidence is far from conclusive, but there has been some controversy about the long-term safety of black cohosh, because of claims of a possible link with liver problems. As a precaution, you should perhaps avoid use if you suffer from liver disease, or if you notice any signs of liver damage (tiredness, loss of appetite, yellowing of skin and eyes, stomach pain with nausea and vomiting, dark urine). You should also check with your GP or pharmacist before taking black cohosh if you take a prescribed medication, such as amiodarone or carbamazepine, which could have a toxic effect on the liver when taken in combination with the black cohosh.

Dong quai

Dong quai is a herb native to China, where it's widely used for gynaecological problems and as a female tonic. It's claimed to reduce hot flushes and vaginal dryness and improve mood, but there's little clinical evidence of its effectiveness. Traditional Chinese herbalists argue that the dong quai works synergistically, so it's more effective when combined with other herbs. A placebo-controlled randomised trial of a dong quai-and-camomile combination seemed to back this up when it found it to be significantly more effective than a placebo in reducing hot flushes.

Dong quai can increase the tendency to bleed, so avoid using it with anti-coagulant drugs such as warfarin. It can also increase sensitivity to sunlight and affect the actions of some drugs, e.g. antidepressants and corticosteroids.

Evening primrose and starflower (borage) oils

Evening primrose and starflower oils are often recommended for reducing hot flushes, night sweats and other menopausal symptoms. They contain a type of omega-6 essential fatty acid called gamma linoleic acid (GLA). Omega-6 fatty acids are vital for various processes in the body, including reproduction. We produce GLA in our bodies from another fatty acid called linoleic acid found in sunflower and corn oils, but only in small amounts, hence supplementation may be beneficial.

There's little evidence that these oils help hot flushes during the day, but there is some suggesting they may cut night sweats. However, one study showed evening primrose oil was no better than a placebo for the relief of flushes and night sweats. There is also some evidence these oils can help ease breast pain and tenderness and prevent mood swings. It is thought that GLA helps to reduce the body's inflammatory response to hormone fluctuations.

Fennel

Both the plant and the seeds appear to have a beneficial effect on progesterone levels in the body. Its aniseed flavour adds interest to food. It can be eaten raw – slice it finely and add it to salads, or roast it in olive oil as a flavoursome accompaniment to chicken. Remove the tough outer layer first. Fennels seeds go well with oily fish, such as mackerel, salmon and herrings. Alternatively, try drinking Twinings Pure Fennel – a herbal infusion made from fennel seeds.

Note: fennel isn't recommended for anyone with epilepsy.

Ginkgo biloba

Studies suggest that this herb, extracted from the maidenhair tree in China, may help with memory problems and ease the 'foggy-headedness' that some women experience during the menopause. It is thought to work by boosting blood flow to the brain.

Note: ginkgo biloba reduces blood clotting so it shouldn't be taken alongside blood-thinning drugs such as warfarin, ibuprofen and aspirin, and should be stopped at least two weeks before scheduled surgery.

Ginseng

Ginseng is a herb native to Korea and China. It's commonly used to help people deal with stress. It's thought to act as an adaptogen – which means it helps balance hormones by acting on the adrenal glands. There's evidence it can boost well-being and reduce depression during and after the menopause.

A few cases of postmenopausal bleeding have been recorded in connection with taking ginseng, as well as interactions with alcohol, warfarin and some antidepressants.

Liquorice root

Liquorice root is the second most prescribed herb in Chinese herbal medicine and North Americans have traditionally used it for menstrual and childbirth problems. It contains two less common types of phytoestrogens – triterpenoids and coumarins – and is thought to have a balancing effect on female hormones. However, there's currently no scientific – just anecdotal – evidence to demonstrate its effectiveness.

Note: the German Commission E warns pregnant women, those with liver or kidney disorders and those taking corticosteroid drugs or cyclosporin against using liquorice root. It contains a substance called glycyrrhizin, which in large amounts can cause high blood pressure, but you can buy products containing 'deglycyrrhizinated liquorice' (DGL) which have had the glycyrrhizin removed.

Maca

Maca is a Peruvian herb known for over three thousand years and thought to stimulate the pituitary gland to produce sex hormones. It's believed to boost energy by stimulating the adrenal glands, as well as reduce menopausal symptoms. In

Peru, where around only two per cent of women take HRT, its widely used to boost libido and reduce hot flushes. There's little scientific evidence to support these claims, but maca is rich in phytonutrients, minerals, amino acids and fatty acids and as such may be worth taking as a general tonic.

Parsley

Parsley contains phytoestrogens. Taken regularly, it can ease menopausal symptoms. Drinking a parsley infusion is reported to relieve cystitis. Pour boiling water over 10 g (two teaspoons) of fresh parsley, or 5 g (one teaspoon) of dried. Cover and leave to stand for 10 minutes. Strain and sweeten with honey if required. Drink whilst hot.

Red clover

This fairly common little wild flower has recently aroused a lot of interest because of its high isoflavone content. Like soya, it contains all four types of isoflavone, and as a result is thought to reduce hot flushes as well as slow down bone loss in postmenopausal women. Some studies have concluded that red clover reduces the frequency of flushes by up to 50 per cent and the severity by up to 44 per cent. However, others report no benefits – this may be because some women can't metabolise phytoestrogens.

Sage

Drink sage tea. Sage is a member of the mint family, traditionally chewed or drunk as tea by Mediterranean women to relieve menopausal symptoms. It seems to be mildly oestrogenic and has an astringent, anti-perspirant effect, making it effective in reducing hot flushes and night sweats. The German Commission

E approves the use of sage for excessive perspiration. You can grow sage in your garden, or buy it as a growing herb at the supermarket. To make sage tea, pour boiling water on three or four freshly picked leaves or one teaspoon of dried sage. You can also add sage to stews and casseroles.

Alternatively, take 15 drops of sage tincture (try Menosan by Bioforce) in water. In a clinical trial, Menosan was shown to half the number of flushes women experienced. Sage has also been traditionally used to enhance memory. Studies show it helps protect levels of acetylcholine, a brain chemical implicated in memory and learning, hence it may help to prevent Alzheimer's. If you dislike the taste of sage, you can take 400 mg daily in tablet or capsule form.

Ayurvedic answers
Shatavari, meaning 'she who has one hundred husbands', is an Indian herb used in Ayurvedic medicine as a female tonic. It's thought to balance hormones, cooling hot flushes and boosting mood and energy levels. Studies using animals have demonstrated its adaptogenic properties. You can buy Shatavari and Shatavari Plus, a product also containing agnus castus, rose, turmeric, ginger, sarsaparilla and other Ayurvedic herbs from Pukka Herbs at www.pukkaherbs.com. This company also produces Harmonise Tea, a herbal tea blending Shatavari, rose flower, vanilla, camomile and hibiscus, which is claimed to assist and support women's health.

St John's wort
St John's wort, often known as 'nature's Prozac' is widely used for its anti-depressant qualities and may be worth trying if you suffer from low mood during the menopause. Research shows this herb

is as effective as mild anti-depressants for the treatment of mild to moderate depression. It's thought to work by increasing levels of brain chemicals linked to mood, including serotonin.

Note: if you're taking any kind of medication, speak to your GP or pharmacist before using St John's wort as it can react with several commonly prescribed drugs, including anti-epileptic drugs, warfarin and the antibiotic tetracycline. It can also increase sensitivity to sunlight.

Tarragon

A tea made from tarragon is reputed to have calming and sedative properties which help to promote sleep.

5-HTP

5-Hydroxytryptophan – 5-HTP – is the precursor to the 'happy chemical' serotonin and is recommended if you suffer from depression, or sleep problems. Clinical studies suggest 5-HTP is as effective as Prozac in treating depression, with fewer side effects. It appears to boost mood by increasing levels of serotonin and aid sleep by raising levels of the sleep-inducing hormone melatonin. Supplements containing 5-HTP are usually made from the seeds of the *Griffonia* plant, from West Africa.

35 Take supplements

Eating a healthy diet containing lots of phytoestrogen-rich foods, taking plenty of exercise and managing your stress levels should always be your main focus for easing menopausal symptoms. However, herb and vitamin combinations allow you to take a range of ingredients in a convenient form. Some studies show that such formulas may be helpful in reducing menopausal symptoms, though there is some controversy over supplementing with vitamins and minerals, as some experts argue that we should obtain the recommended nutrients from our diets. My feelings are that it is best to eat a healthy diet containing all of the essential nutrients, but for various reasons not everyone manages to do this, so sometimes a vitamin and/or mineral supplement might be beneficial. The following list details some of the commercial formulations currently available, with an overview of the main ingredients and possible benefits.

Boots Menopause Support Plus – multivitamins and minerals with soya isoflavones, sage, green tea, flaxseed and PABA. The isoflavones could help reduce flushes and strengthen bones. The sage and flaxseed may also ease hot flushes and night sweats.

Emerita Pro-Gest – a 'natural' progesterone cream which is massaged into the skin. Nutritional therapist Marilyn Glenville argues that after the menopause your body no longer needs progesterone, so if you stop producing it, why take it? She also points out that whilst it's produced from diosgenin from wild yams, the chemical processes involved mean it's not 'natural'. However, in clinical trials women using progesterone cream suffered from fewer hot flushes, so if nothing else has worked for you, it may be worth a try.

MenoCool – contains hops, the isoflavones genisteine and daidzein, buckwheat, black oats, malt, barley, rye and wheat. The various ingredients provide a mix of isoflavones that could help balance hormones and reduce symptoms such as flushing.

Meno-Herbs 2 – wild yam root, black cohosh root, red clover leaf, dong quai root, raspberry, vitex agnus castus, Siberian ginseng, partridge berry, nettle leaf and grapeseed extract. Another herbal combination that could help balance hormones, reduce flushing and improve mood and energy levels.

Menolife Day and Night – the day formula contains calcium and magnesium, soya bean extract, dong quai, black cohosh, red clover extract, wild yam extract, chaste tree extract (agnus castus), St John's wort and Siberian ginseng root. The night formula is the same, except the St John's wort and Siberian ginseng are replaced by valerian root and passiflora to aid sleep. This mix of herbs could help reduce hot flushes and other menopausal symptoms, as well as boost mood and protect bone health.

MenoMood St John's Wort extract 300 mg and Black Cohosh root extract 6.4 mg – a study in 2006 noted that black cohosh and St John's wort work well together to reduce both psychological and physical menopausal symptoms. This herbal medicine has been registered under the Traditional Herbal Registration (THR) scheme, a regulatory approval process for herbal treatments in the EU. This means it meets specific standards of safety and quality, based on traditional usage.

Menopace – vitamin B complex, zinc, magnesium, vitamins A, C, D and E and soya isoflavone extract. This formulation could reduce stress, boost bone and heart health and reduce menopausal symptoms such as flushing.

Menopace Plus – contains the original tablets, plus 'active botanical' tablets, which contain extra soya isoflavones, flaxseed lignans, sage extract and green tea extract. These may help to provide additional support during the menopause.

Novogen Red Clover – contains a standardised 40 mg of isoflavones from red clover, which could help to reduce the frequency and severity of hot flushes.

Promensil – a range of products containing a natural standardised extract of red clover isoflavones. The original formula contains 40 mg of isoflavones, while the double strength contains 80 mg. There is also a postmenopausal formula which contains calcium and vitamin D3 to help promote bone and heart health.

Vitamin C-1000 with Bioflavonoids Caplets 1000 mg (Holland & Barrett) – taking vitamin C with bioflavonoids in tablet form has been shown to reduce the incidence of hot flushes. Bioflavonoids are thought to be similar in structure to oestrogen. Vitamin C also aids the functioning of the adrenal glands, which produce androstenedione, the precursor to oestrone.

Ymea – a combination of soya, hops and bitter melon. Isoflavones from the soya and hops could reduce flushing and may help protect against osteoporosis. Bitter melon contains antioxidants, which can reduce visible signs of ageing.

Chapter 5

More Hints for a Healthier Menopause

This section offers practical tips to help you reduce your risk of developing any of the three main lady-killers linked to the menopause – cardiovascular disease, breast cancer and osteoporosis. There are also details of risk factors, as well as simple health checks that can help to detect increased risk, or early signs of disease. Plus, you'll find suggestions to help you deal with other health problems associated with the menopause, including migraine, cystitis, incontinence and insomnia.

Take heart

Research shows that going through the menopause more than doubles your risk of developing cardiovascular disease, a collective term for heart and artery diseases i.e. coronary heart disease and stroke, which is caused by atherosclerosis. Atherosclerosis, or hardening of the arteries, stems from a build-up of fatty deposits (LDL cholesterol) in the artery walls. This is thought to be due in part to falling levels of oestrogen. Oestrogen is believed to protect the heart and reduce 'bad' LDL cholesterol levels during the child-bearing years. But lifestyle also plays an important part. The main risks are a stressful lifestyle, smoking, heavy drinking, a poor diet, weight gain – especially around the middle, and a sedentary lifestyle.

Ask your GP or practice nurse to check your cholesterol level. It's a good idea to have your blood pressure checked regularly too, as it's thought to be responsible for around half of all coronary heart disease. The British Heart Foundation offers more detailed advice on keeping your heart healthy – the contact details are in the directory at the end of this book.

36 Walk your way to health

A study at the University of Applied Sciences in Tampere, Finland, in 2015 found that 49-year-old women who took regular exercise had a better quality of life and fewer menopausal symptoms such as hot flushes, insomnia, anxiety, depression, and memory and concentration problems. Being active may reduce flushes because it helps to control stress. Also, the endorphins (feel-good chemicals) your body releases during exercise are responsible for the psychological benefits. Exercise will also help you control your weight at a time when hormones are conspiring to pile the fat around your middle.

You don't need to go to the gym – walking is a great form of exercise that you can fit into your everyday routine. Walking lowers the risk of other health problems linked to the postmenopause; it increases cardiovascular fitness and reduces blood pressure, cholesterol and body fat, thus lowering the risk of strokes and heart attacks. Because walking is a weight-bearing exercise, it wards off osteoporosis by stimulating your bones to maintain a stronger structure. Walking and other forms of exercise have also been proven to slow down mental decline associated with age. Regular walking reduces the risk of developing breast and colon cancers, type 2 diabetes, and strengthens your muscles, as well as helping prevent 'middle-age spread' – and it costs you nothing.

Ways to walk more

Park your car further from the office or the shops, or leave the car at home if they are within walking distance. Walk up and down the platform, rather than standing still, whilst waiting for the train. Do the same at the bus stand. Get off the bus or train one stop earlier – though of course do this only during daylight hours and avoid isolated areas. Take a 15-minute walk during your lunch break, rather than sitting at your desk. For short trips, leave the car and walk. Walk as you talk on your cordless, or mobile phone.

Walking for Health is a national body offering information, support and encouragement to complete beginners, existing walkers and health and leisure professionals (see Directory).

Canine trainer

Get a dog, or offer to walk your neighbour's, and you'll benefit from having your own personal canine fitness trainer! Research shows that dog owners take more exercise and are fitter than gym members. On average, a dog owner walks 676 miles each year, compared to 468 miles for a gym-goer. Dog owners also enjoy slightly lower blood pressure. When you have a dog you tend to take more exercise because you have to exercise your pet 'come rain or shine', whereas gym members are more likely to stay at home when the weather is bad.

37 Be breast aware

Being breast aware involves knowing how your breasts normally feel and being aware of the changes to look out for. Breast Cancer Care, a UK charity which provides information, practical assistance and emotional support to those affected by breast cancer, currently advises that there's no set way to check your breasts, but you should aim to do so regularly, following this five point code:

1. Know what's normal for you

2. Know what changes to look and feel for

3. Look and feel

4. Report any changes to your GP without delay

5. Attend routine breast screening if you're aged 50 or over

Changes to be aware of:

- Size – if one breast becomes larger, or lower

- Nipples – if a nipple becomes inverted (pulled in) or changes position or shape

- Rashes – on or around the nipple

- Discharge – from one or both nipples

- Skin changes – puckering or dimpling

- Swelling – under the armpit or around the collarbone

- Pain – continuous, in one part of the breast or armpit

- A lump or thickening – different to the rest of the breast tissue

If you detect a change in your breasts, try not to worry – most changes aren't cancer, but visit your GP as soon as you can. The contact details for Breast Cancer Care and also Cancer Research UK are in the directory at the end of this book.

Breast cancer – the risks

We've already looked at some of the risk factors for breast cancer: taking HRT for five years or longer can increase the risk slightly, as can drinking alcohol – the more you drink, the higher the risk. There is no need to abstain – the advice is to drink within the government's lower risk guidelines, which is no more than 2–3 units daily. For further information on alcohol and your health, go to the Drinkaware website – details of which are in the directory at the back of the book. Other factors include:

- Age – the older you are, the greater your risk.

- The contraceptive pill – slightly increases risk, but returns to normal gradually after you stop taking it.

- Being overweight.

- Having a close family member diagnosed with breast cancer increases your risk – but in nine out of ten cases there's no family history of the disease.

- Early menstruation and late menopause – the longer you have periods, the greater your risk.

- The more children you have and the younger you are when you have them, reduces your risk, as does breastfeeding.

- As is the case for osteoporosis and cardiovascular disease, a healthy diet and being physically active can reduce your risk of developing breast cancer.

38 Manage migraines

If you suffer from migraines, you may find they increase during the menopause due to hormonal changes. Following the suggestions on managing stress and natural HRT may help to reduce their frequency, but if they continue despite your best efforts the following tips may help.

- Try taking feverfew tablets daily. Research has shown that this herb is effective in preventing migraines. Alternatively, you can try fresh feverfew leaves. The leaves are bitter, so try a couple daily in a honey sandwich. You can buy a feverfew plant and keep it outdoors.

- Try taking 200 mg magnesium tablets twice daily. Studies have shown magnesium can help to prevent migraines.

- There's also evidence that vitamin B12 (riboflavin) can reduce the number of migraines sufferers experience. Good sources of vitamin B12 include wholemeal bread, liver, low-fat milk and yogurt, mackerel and eggs.

- 5-HTP – a supplement mentioned in chapter 4 – may also help reduce migraines if they're due to low levels of serotonin, the hormone linked to mood.

- Melatonin, the hormone that regulates sleep, is another supplement that has been shown to help migraines – as well as improve sleep patterns. Research suggests there is a link between sleep patterns and migraine; many migraine sufferers find that too much or too little sleep is a migraine trigger. Also, it appears that we produce less melatonin as we get older. The recommended dosage is 3 mg every night, half an hour before bed.

- If you feel a migraine coming on, take a suitable painkiller as soon as you can. Some sufferers find analgesics such as ibuprofen, aspirin or paracetamol work quite well. Others need to take a drug specifically aimed at treating migraines such as 5HT 1 receptor agonists, which work by reducing the size of the blood vessels around the brain – it's believed that the temporary swelling of these blood vessels may be the cause of migraine symptoms. These drugs are available on prescription and over the counter at pharmacies. However, taking too many painkillers can increase the number of migraines.

- Drinking coffee or cola can help to abort a migraine. (Though cola shouldn't be drunk often, as it has a detrimental effect on the bones – see 'Keep your bones healthy' in chapter 4.) The caffeine they contain is thought to maximise the effectiveness of painkillers and may also help to constrict the blood vessels around the brain. However, too much caffeine can trigger migraines.

- Lie down in a quiet and darkened room either with a cool gel pack or a heated pad – whichever works for you.

- Chew raw ginger or drink peppermint tea to ease the nausea. Evidence suggests that ginger may also prevent attacks by blocking the effects of prostaglandins – substances which can inflame blood vessels in the brain, leading to migraine.

39 Stop cystitis

To prevent cystitis, wear underwear made from cotton rather than synthetic fibres, and avoid thongs, which can introduce bacteria from the back passage into the vagina.

Apply natural yogurt to the vagina to relieve the stinging and burning sensation of cystitis. Adding about 50 ml of vinegar to your bath helps to restore the pH balance and curbs bacterial growth. Alternatively, add about six drops of camomile oil to a warm bath to soothe away stinging and irritation. Tea tree oil can be added to the bath, or used in a douche. To make a douche add two drops of oil to 5 ml (one teaspoon) of vodka, then dilute the mixture with one pint of boiled, cooled water. Some women suffer from cystitis symptoms without the infection. This is usually caused by atrophy of the vaginal tissues and vaginal oestrogen cream is often the only way to treat it effectively – see your GP. For more information on what to eat and drink to prevent cystitis, see 'Eat to ease cystitis' in chapter 4. If your symptoms persist, or you experience blood in your urine, chills, nausea, vomiting, or lower back pain, always seek medical help.

40 Beat incontinence

Urinary incontinence is an involuntary loss of urine. Around one in five women in their 50s are thought to suffer from it. Falling oestrogen levels may be to blame, along with age, childbearing, hysterectomy and being overweight.

Pelvic floor exercises can help in 75 per cent of cases. An easy exercise is to stop the stream for just a second halfway through urinating. You can also try tightening the vaginal, bottom and pelvic floor muscles upwards and inwards whenever you're sitting down. The Bladder and Bowel Foundation offers more information and advice (see Directory).

41 Sleep more soundly

In a recent survey, eight out of ten menopausal women claimed to suffer from disturbed sleep. Some women have no problem falling asleep, but night sweats wake them during the night and they find it difficult to drop off again. Obviously, you need to take steps to deal with the hot flushes first (see 'Sleep tight' in chapter 2), but if you still have problems sleeping, here are a few strategies you can try.

- Get out during the day. Exposure to sunlight halts the production of sleep-inducing melatonin and promotes its release at night.

- Make sure your bedroom is cool (around 16 ºC) and dark. A reduced body temperature slows the metabolism, making waking from hunger less likely. Darkness stimulates the production of melatonin.

- Don't keep a TV or computer in the bedroom. Watching TV or using a computer last thing at night can overstimulate your brain, and the bright lights from both may inhibit the production of melatonin.

- Avoid drinking coffee or cola after 2 p.m., as the stimulant effects of the caffeine they contain can last for hours. Whilst tea contains around half as much caffeine – around 50 mg per cup – it's best not to overdo it near bedtime. Try drinking rooibos tea, which is caffeine free, instead.

- Avoid alcohol – although it may relax you initially and help you fall asleep more quickly, it has a stimulant effect, causing you to wake more during the night. It's also a diuretic, making night-time trips to the toilet more likely.

- If abstinence from alcohol brings no improvement, a glass of Cabernet Sauvignon, Merlot or Chianti at bedtime could improve your sleep patterns, because they're rich in the sleep hormone melatonin.

- Being inactive all day can cause restlessness and sleep problems. Exercise can help you sleep more soundly, because it causes your body temperature and metabolism to rise and then fall a few hours later, which encourages sleep. To benefit, don't exercise any later than early evening.

- Choose foods rich in tryptophan, an amino acid your body uses to produce serotonin – a brain chemical which induces sleepiness. Tryptophan-rich foods include bananas, chicken, turkey, dates, rice, oats, wholegrain breads and cereals.

- Make sure you're neither too hungry nor too full when you go to bed, as both can cause wakefulness.

- Soak in a warm bath at bedtime. The heat raises your temperature slightly and the temperature drop that follows encourages sleep. Add a few drops of lavender or camomile essential oils for their relaxing properties.

- If worrying about problems or a busy schedule the next day keeps you awake, try writing down your concerns or a plan for the next day before you go to bed.

Cope with the change the Chinese way

Studies show that acupuncture can help with various menopausal symptoms, including hot flushes, anxiety, depression and general aches and pains. It's been used in Chinese medicine for over 5,000 years and involves inserting fine needles into the skin to stimulate 'acupoints' to allow the flow of qi or life force through the body. It's believed that endorphins – the body's natural painkillers – are released when the needles puncture the acupoints. Research also suggests that acupuncture can increase the levels of oestrogen in the body. Acupuncture is not something you could try at home. You should consult a qualified practitioner. To find a qualified, registered acupuncturist near you contact the British Acupuncture Council (see Directory for details). Acupressure is described as 'acupuncture without needles'. For acupressure techniques you could try for yourself, see chapter 6.

Chapter 6

DIY Complementary Therapies

The main difference between complementary therapies, often also known as alternative, natural or holistic therapies, and conventional Western medicine, is that the former approach focusses on treating the individual as a whole, whereas the latter is symptom led. Complementary practitioners view illness as a sign that physical and mental well-being have been disrupted and attempt to restore good health by stimulating the body's own self-healing and self-regulating abilities. They claim that total well-being can be achieved when the mind and body are in a state of balance called homeostasis. Homeostasis is achieved by following the type of lifestyle advocated in this book, i.e. a healthy diet and plenty of fresh air, exercise, sleep and relaxation, combined with stress management and a positive mental attitude.

Unlike drug treatments, which are comparatively recent, complementary therapies like aromatherapy, massage and reflexology have been used to treat ailments and promote well-being for thousands of years.

In this chapter you'll find a brief overview of complementary therapies that could boost your well-being during the menopause and beyond, along with simple techniques and treatments for particular symptoms that you could try for yourself at home.

42 Apply acupressure

Acupressure is part of traditional Chinese medicine and is often referred to as 'acupuncture without needles'. Like acupuncture, it's based on the idea that life energy, or qi, flows through channels in the body known as meridians. An even passage of qi throughout the body is viewed as necessary to good health. Disruption of the flow of qi in a meridian can lead to illness at any point along it. The flow of qi can be affected by various lifestyle factors, including stress, emotional distress, diet and environment.

Qi is the most concentrated at points along the meridians known as acupoints. Using the fingers to apply firm but gentle pressure to these points stimulates the body's natural self-healing abilities. Muscle tension is relieved and the circulation boosted, thereby promoting good health. The application of pressure also seems to stimulate the production of endorphins – the body's natural painkillers. Studies confirm the benefits of stimulating acupoints. Research shows that applying pressure to an acupoint 5 cm above the wrist crease nearest the hand relieves nausea. The stimulation of acupoints using acupressure has proved effective for treating alcohol addiction and back and neck pain.

Alleviate anxiety with acupressure

It's claimed that applying pressure to two acupoints on your feet can help alleviate anxiety and insomnia during the menopause.

Using the middle and index fingers of your left hand, press firmly on the indentation below your ankle bone on the inside of your right ankle for 1 to 3 minutes. Repeat using your right hand for your left ankle.

Next, using the middle and index fingers of your right hand, press on the indentation on the outside of your right ankle, just below the ankle bone for 1 to 3 minutes. Repeat with your left hand on your left ankle.

43 Use aroma power

Essential oils are extracted by various methods from the petals, leaves, stalk, roots, seeds, nuts and even the bark of plants. Aromatherapy is based on the belief that when scents released from essential oils are inhaled, they affect the hypothalamus, the part of the brain which regulates the glands and hormones, altering mood and lowering stress levels. When used in massage, baths and compresses, the oils are also absorbed through the skin into the bloodstream and transported to the organs and glands, which benefit from their healing effects. A couple of studies have suggested that essential oils such as neroli, valerian and lavender can aid relaxation and induce calm. During a small study in 2005, participants with menopausal symptoms who used aromatherapy oils and massage reported an improvement in their physical and mental health.

Essentials oils are highly concentrated and generally need to be diluted in a carrier oil such as almond, wheatgerm or grapeseed to prevent skin irritation. Always buy the best quality oils you can afford. That said, good quality olive, sunflower or sesame oils from your kitchen will work well – especially if they're organic. The recommended concentration of essential oils is no more than 2.5 per cent for adults. One teaspoon (5 ml) of carrier oil equals 100 drops. So as a rough guide, add two drops of essential oil per 5 ml of carrier oil. You'll find aromatherapy oils at most high street chemists. Tisserand Aromatherapy and Natural by Nature Oils offer a wide range of good quality essential oils – contact details for both are in the directory.

Antidepressant oils

Depression is a problem for some women during the menopause. A number of essential oils are recommended for their anti-depressant qualities. These include bergamot, rose, clary sage, jasmine, ylang-ylang, neroli, lavender and sandalwood.

Coming up roses

As an all-round booster for during the menopause, rose oil is hard to beat. With its delicate aroma and mood-lifting, hormone-balancing and beautifying effects, it can help promote feelings of femininity and beat menopausal symptoms as oestrogen levels decline. It's thought to help tone and cleanse the uterus, as well as comfort, lift the spirits and act as an aphrodisiac. It's also great for ageing skin, having toning, soothing and moisturising properties. It soothes sensitive skin and helps to reduce the redness associated with 'thread veins'.

Cypress oil

Cypress oil is recommended to help alleviate heavy bleeding. Although heavy bleeding can be linked to the menopause, if it's a persistent problem, you should consult your GP to check there are no other underlying causes.

Hormone-balancing oils

Geranium oil is a hormone balancer. Clary sage, fennel, tarragon and star anise oils have oestrogenic effects, making them useful as your body adapts to lower oestrogen levels. Clary sage also has antiperspirant properties and may help to reduce hot flushes and night sweats. It's also an aphrodisiac.

Note: fennel oil is not recommended for anyone with epilepsy.

Lavender relaxer

For speedy stress relief, sniff lavender. It contains linalool, which is thought to stimulate brain receptors for GABA (Gamma-aminobutyric acid), a brain chemical that induces calm. Inhaling for 5 minutes also reduces the stress hormone cortisol.

Menopause mixture

Rose, geranium, clary sage and lavender oils blend well together. For a balanced oil that will help ease menopausal symptoms such as anxiety, depression, flushing and low libido, add three drops of each to 25 ml of carrier oil. Use as a massage oil, or add to the bath.

Camomile calm

Try Roman camomile oil, either for massage or in the bath, for relief from several menopause symptoms. Roman camomile oil is claimed to ease pain, soothe and calm, thus aiding sleep and reducing flushes and mood swings. Alternatively, drink camomile tea for similar benefits.

Anti-wrinkle massage

An aromatherapy facial massage can help prevent and treat wrinkles. Massage stimulates the nerve endings, helping to tighten and tone the skin to give a natural facelift. The most beneficial time to do this is before you go to bed, so that you can leave the oils on the skin overnight.

Add two drops of rose, frankincense, neroli or patchouli essential oil to 5 ml (one teaspoon) of a moisturising base oil, such as wheatgerm, jojoba, or peach kernel. The Egyptians used frankincense not only for embalming but also for cosmetic purposes because of its ability to preserve the skin. Neroli and patchouli both stimulate skin cell renewal.

Method: pour the oil into the palms and rub together. Apply the oil with both hands, using long, upward and outward strokes, to the neck, cheeks, nose and forehead. Next, using your fingertips, tap all over the face and neck to stimulate the circulation. Finish by massaging all over with gentle, circular movements.

44 Use flower power

Flower essences have been used for their healing properties for thousands of years. However, it was Dr Edward Bach, a Harley Street doctor, bacteriologist and homeopath, who developed their use in the twentieth century. Bach identified 38 basic negative states of mind and devised a plant or flower-based remedy for each. The remedies are thought to help counteract negative emotions, such as despair, fear and uncertainty, but there's only anecdotal evidence regarding their effectiveness. They're widely available in pharmacies in handbag-sized 10- and 20-ml phials.

Bach Rescue Remedy is designed to help you cope with times of acute stress and may help with hot flushes. Other Bach remedies that may be appropriate include Scleranthus for mood swings, Mustard for melancholy and Walnut for periods of transition. For further information on how to select a suitable flower remedy and an online questionnaire which enables you to select a personalised blend, visit www.bachfloweressences.co.uk.

45 Get homeopathic healing

Homeopathy is based on the theory that 'like cures like': substances that can cause symptoms in a well person can treat the same symptoms in an ill person and encourage the body to heal itself. The substances used in homeopathic remedies come from plant, animal, metal and mineral sources that are made into a tincture, which is then diluted many times. Homeopaths claim that the more diluted a remedy is, the higher its potency and the lower its potential side effects. They claim that through the 'memory of water' molecules from substances that are diluted away leave behind an electromagnetic 'footprint' – rather like a recording on an audio tape – which has an effect on the body.

Whilst the jury is still out regarding its efficacy, some research suggests it can help alleviate menopausal symptoms. It's best to consult a trained homeopath, who will recommend a remedy based on your particular symptoms, and your physical, mental and emotional state. However, you can buy homeopathic remedies at many high street pharmacies. There are over 150 homeopathic remedies which could help alleviate menopausal symptoms. The following list includes the most widely recommended. If you're buying over the counter, select the remedy indicated for the range of symptoms that most closely match the ones you're experiencing. In his book, *Encyclopedia of Homeopathy*, the late renowned homeopath Dr Andrew Lockie recommends 30 c (1:100 dilution carried out 30 times) of the appropriate remedy twice daily for up to seven days at a time to treat menopausal symptoms. The remedies are usually available in 6 c and 30 c potencies.

Belladonna – prescribed for insomnia, excitability, restlessness and an overactive mind.

Calcarea carbonica – suggested for an inability to cope emotionally with the menopause, headache that's worse on the left side, perspiration on the face and back of the neck during sleep and a craving for sweet foods.

Lycopodium clavatum – is recommended for physical weakness accompanied by a sharp mind. Also recommended for people who tend to wake up in the early hours and are then unable to drop back off to sleep because they start mulling things over.

Sanguinaria canadensis – also known as bloodroot – is thought to ease most menopausal symptoms, including hot flushes, night sweats, breast soreness, unpleasant vaginal discharges and heavy menstrual bleeding.

Lachesis mutus – also helps with flushes and sweats, nervous irritability and anxiety, ovarian pain, migraines and palpitations.

Pulsatilla – is recommended for the treatment of flushes which mainly occur indoors. Also for moodiness and feeling weepy.

Sepia – is used for womb problems such as prolapse, a dragging feeling in the abdomen, vaginal dryness, thrush infections, sudden hot flushes and loss of libido.

Nux vomica – helps the body to adjust to reduced oestrogen levels. Particularly used for night sweats that lead to chills.

Valeriana – is recommended for flushes which mainly affect the face and cause extreme sweating.

Amyl nitrosum – used for flushes affecting the face, especially if accompanied by throbbing in the head, and heavy sweating. Also for anxiety and palpitations.

Sulphur – is suggested for women who suffer from heat sensitivity and night sweats that cause thirstiness.

46 Find relief in reflexology

The philosophy underpinning reflexology is similar to that of acupuncture and acupressure. Reflexology is based on the idea that points on the feet, hands and face, known as reflexes, correspond to different parts of the body (e.g. glands and organs). These are linked via vertical zones, along which energy flows and illness occurs when these zones become blocked. Stimulating the reflexes using the fingers and thumbs is thought to bring about physiological changes, which remove these blockages and encourage the mind and body to self-heal.

Practitioners believe that imbalances in the body result in granular deposits in the relevant reflex, which cause tenderness. Corns, bunions and even hard skin are thought to indicate problems in the relevant parts of the body. Medical opinion is divided. One trial showed that ordinary foot massage reduced menopausal symptoms equally as well as refexology. However, there's anecdotal evidence that reflexology may help and foot massage is relaxing and stress-relieving.

DIY reflexology

It's usually easier to apply reflexology to your hands and face than to your own feet, so the following techniques focus on these areas. For extra stimulation, use a small rotating movement in the direction of your spine.

Work your adrenal reflexes

Healthy adrenal gland function is vital during and after the menopause. To stimulate the adrenals, use the thumb of the opposite hand to apply firm pressure to the point between the thumb and forefinger, a couple of centimetres into the palm. Hold for a few seconds. Repeat three times on each palm.

Stimulate your womb reflexes

To stimulate your womb reflex and encourage your womb to function efficiently – especially during the perimenopause – use the middle finger of your other hand to apply firm pressure to the outside edge of your wrist below the thumb. Hold for a few seconds. Repeat three times on each wrist.

Activate your ovary reflexes

Activating these reflexes could help to keep your hormones balanced. Using the middle finger of your other hand, apply pressure to the area just in front of your wrist bone, below your little finger. Hold for a few seconds and repeat three times.

Facial reflexology

A woman suffering from up to thirty flushes a day recently claimed that her symptoms diminished to a couple a day after just two facial reflexology treatments. By the fifth they'd all but disappeared.

Draw an imaginary line from where each eyebrow ends down to each cheekbone. The reproductive system facial reflex points are situated on each cheekbone, midway between this point and the beginning of your ear. Using the tips of your index fingers, simultaneously massage both reflexes with small, gentle, circular movements in an outward direction.

47 Say 'yes' to yoga

The word yoga comes from the Sanskrit word *yuj*, which means union. Yogic postures and breathing exercises are designed to unite the body, mind and soul. It's a gentle form of exercise which not only strengthens and increases flexibility but also induces calm and relieves stress as well as aches and pains. Yoga poses help to balance the endocrine system, which controls hormone production and the heart rate. The postures are weight-bearing, helping to prevent osteoporosis. Inverted postures, such as the shoulder stand, boost circulation and blood flow to the upper body, helping to increase alertness and improve the health of skin and hair. Yoga is also believed to benefit the nervous system, aid weight-control and tone and firm the muscles. Yoga breathing techniques increase oxygen in the blood and studies suggest they can cut asthma attacks, migraines, irritable bowel syndrome (IBS) and other conditions.

In a nutshell, yoga can improve your mind, body and appearance, making it a great form of exercise during the menopause and beyond. The best way to learn yoga is by attending classes run by a qualified teacher. To find one near you, go to The British Wheel of Yoga's website – www.bwy.org.uk. Or, if you'd prefer to teach yourself at home, visit www.abc-of-yoga.com, a site which shows you how to do the various postures and even suggests a basic yoga routine to follow during the menopause.

When practising yoga at home always proceed gently and avoid forcing your body into postures. Always stop if you feel any discomfort. Wear lightweight, loose clothing to allow you to move freely and no footwear, as yoga is best performed barefoot. Use a non-slip mat if the floor is slippery. Don't attempt inverted postures if you have a neck or back problem, or have high blood pressure, heart disease or circulatory problems. If in doubt, consult your GP first.

Cooling yoga breath

This is said to be both cooling and relaxing – ideal for when a hot flush strikes. Curl your tongue to resemble a tube, allowing the tip to stick out slightly. If you find this too difficult, or you're using the technique in public, simply keep your mouth slightly open so that the air passes over your tongue. Breathe in slowly and deeply through the mouth. The air should feel cool as it passes over your tongue. Keeping your tongue in the same position, breathe out slowly and deeply through the mouth. Repeat several times and you should experience a cooling effect.

Chapter 7

Look Younger

Many women believe that their femininity is inextricably linked to their fertility, so after the menopause they feel they're somehow less of a woman. Hormonal changes can contribute to weight gain, leave the skin more prone to sagging and wrinkling and the hair may become drier and thinner. Little wonder many women lose confidence in their appearance at this time – in a recent survey four out of ten postmenopausal women said they were 'afraid of their physical appearance'.

But, with a little extra care, it's still possible to look great – whatever your age. Taking care of your looks is not just vanity – knowing you look your best improves your self-image, which in turn increases your self-esteem and confidence. Research suggests that high self-esteem boosts immunity and lowers stress and anxiety. Most of us have experienced the psychological boost of a new hairdo or outfit when we're feeling low.

Managing your weight is important, not only so you can look younger – nothing is more ageing than being overweight – but also from a health perspective.

So go on – take care of yourself. Make sensible food choices and be more active. Make the most of your skin and hair. Choose clothes which emphasise your best features. Enhance your looks with subtle make-up and boost both your mood and confidence with your favourite perfume. Read on for tips to keep you looking and feeling young and feminine well beyond the menopause.

48 Take steps towards younger-looking skin

Oestrogen is involved in skin cell metabolism – lower levels at menopause lead to loss of collagen, the main protein in your skin that gives it strength, elasticity and moisture. Elastin, the other main fibrous protein which gives skin its 'bounce' also decreases. As a result the skin becomes thinner, drier and more prone to wrinkling.

The good news is that experts claim that wrinkles are just 30 per cent hereditary and 70 per cent down to lifestyle factors. So there's plenty you can do to slow down the ageing process. I for one think this is preferable to resorting to cosmetic surgery, which can be risky.

Secrets of younger looking skin

The main secrets of younger looking skin are:

- A balanced diet
- Drinking plenty of water
- Sufficient sleep
- Regular exercise
- Not smoking
- Drinking alcohol only in moderation
- Protection from the sun
- Daily cleansing
- Regular exfoliation
- Daily moisturising

The food factor

First and foremost, if you want younger looking skin, you need to feed and moisturise it from the inside. That means ensuring that you eat a balanced diet to provide the vitamins and other nutrients your skin needs to keep healthy.

Eat an ACE diet

Vitamins A, C and E are antioxidants, which means they neutralise the skin-ageing free radicals the body produces when we're stressed, or exposed to sunlight, and pollutants such as cigarette smoke, chemicals and food additives. Vitamin A is also essential for your skin's growth and repair. Vitamin C may boost the production of collagen. Vitamin E keeps your skin soft and smooth from the inside.

Vitamin A comes in two forms – as retinol and beta-carotene. Retinol is found in liver, fish-liver oils, egg yolks, whole milk, cheese and butter. Beta-carotene is found mainly in yellow and orange fruits and vegetables such as carrots, sweet potatoes, butternut squash, cantaloupe melons, orange and yellow peppers and apricots.

Vitamin C is found in fruit and vegetables – particularly citrus fruits, berries, broccoli and cabbage.

Vitamin E is found in nuts and seeds, avocados, sweet potatoes, olive oil and wheatgerm.

Buon appetito!

Eating dishes with tomato-based sauces, such as pasta and pizza, could protect your skin from the damaging effects of the sun. Research suggests that lycopene, an antioxidant in tomatoes which protects the plant from sunlight, may do the same for us. Cooked, rather than raw tomatoes, provide lycopene in its most easily absorbed form, because cooking releases it from the cell walls. Tomato paste is a concentrated source.

In one study, women who ate 55 g (11 teaspoons) of tomato paste – providing 16 mg of lycopene – every day for three months increased their skin's protection from ultra-violet radiation damage by 30 per cent. Lycopene dissolves in fat, so eating cooked tomatoes with a food that contains fat (e.g. cheese or olive oil) helps with absorption. Pastas and pizzas often contain all three, making them a good choice to help prevent skin ageing. For the healthiest versions, choose wholewheat pastas with vegetable or seafood toppings and serve with salad.

Tip: store fresh tomatoes at room temperature, to allow the plant enzymes to produce one fifth more lycopene and double the beta-carotene content. Guavas, pink grapefruits and watermelons also contain lycopene.

Drink green tea
Green tea contains polyphenols – antioxidants thought to protect the skin against sun damage. Evidence suggests you can benefit either by drinking it or by using products containing green tea extracts.

Berry protection
Berries such as raspberries, blueberries, cranberries and strawberries all contain ellagic acid, another antioxidant which boosts the skin's defences against sun damage. Perhaps this is another sign of nature knowing best, seeing as these fruits are in season at the very time of the year when our skin needs the most protection. Pomegranates are also rich in ellagic acid.

Skin-smoothing fats
For soft, smooth, plumped-up skin with few wrinkles, you need to include fats in your diet. Avoid saturated animal fats, which

are linked to hardening of the arteries, coronary heart disease and stroke and eat more omega-3 and omega-6 fatty acids. These oils protect the skin from moisture loss. Good sources of omega-3s include oily fish, such as pilchards, sardines, salmon and mackerel, as well as dark green vegetables, nuts, seeds, egg yolks and linseed (flaxseed), hemp and rapeseed oils. The Perricone Plan, followed by celebrities such as Kim Cattrall, Cate Blanchett, Uma Thurman and Julia Roberts, advocates these foods, claiming they can smooth and lift the skin in days.

Omega-6s, found in sunflower and corn oils, olives, nuts, seeds and whole grains are also essential for healthy skin structure and help maintain its moisture balance.

Go sugar-free

According to Fredric Brandt, dermatologist to Madonna, Cher and Ellen Barkin, cutting sugar from your diet can make your skin look ten years younger. He claims that sugar damages your skin's elastin and collagen, resulting in wrinkling and sagging. Brandt promises that if you cut out, or at least reduce, your intake of sugar-laden cakes, biscuits and sweets, you'll be rewarded with firmer, more toned and radiant skin. Watch out for hidden sugars in processed foods, like tomato sauce. Check food labels – many low-fat products, for example yogurts and cereal bars, are high in sugar. Remember it's not just your skin that could benefit – your waistline could too.

Save the salt

As well as being detrimental to your health – see chapter 4 – too much salt plays havoc with your appearance. It can lead to fluid retention, which manifests itself in puffiness around the eyes and cellulite.

Drink plenty of water

Drinking around 1.2 litres of water daily keeps your skin hydrated and flushes out toxins, to keep your skin plumped-up and clear.

Don't smoke

Smoking reduces the amount of oxygen reaching the skin, making it dull and grey, and increases ageing free radicals in the body. It also leads to deep wrinkling around the mouth and eyes through drawing on a cigarette and squinting to avoid the smoke haze. Smoking also stains the gums and teeth and increases the risk of periodontal disease, which leads to swollen gums and bad breath, as well as causing teeth to fall out. Smoking is also thought to increase hot flushes because it hampers the production of oestrogen.

Sleep on it

Ensuring you get sufficient sleep is important. When you're tired, your skin looks tired too. Sleeping on your back is best – it has been suggested that lying with your face buried in a pillow can cause wrinkles. If menopausal symptoms are affecting your sleep, check out the advice on tackling sleep problems in chapter 5.

Sun protection

UV radiation from the sun damages the elastin and collagen fibres in the skin, causing lasting damage and premature ageing. Most dermatologists agree that the best way to prevent wrinkles is to protect your skin from the sun at all times. Wear a moisturiser or foundation with a minimum sun protection factor of 15 every day. Always apply sun cream to your body prior to exposure and reapply frequently. Choose products with both UVA and UVB protection to protect your body from the ageing and burning effects of the sun. For the best protection experts recommend that we apply sunscreen liberally and don't rub it in too much. Avoid the sun's rays between 10 a.m. and 3 p.m. – this is the time when they are at their strongest. Cover up, or stay in the shade – but remember the sun's rays reflect off water, sand and snow, so still wear protection.

Squeaky clean

Keeping the skin clean is vital. Ageing skin tends to be drier, so avoid using soap or foaming cleansers, which may strip away moisture. Instead, experts recommend using a rinse-off lotion or cream. A clean flannel or muslin cloth rung out in lukewarm water removes the cleanser efficiently and exfoliates gently as well. If you cleanse well at night your skin is unlikely to be dirty next morning – a rinse with cool water may suffice.

Tone up

Alcohol-based toners are best avoided, as they strip away moisture. A facial spritzer containing mineral water or rose water, or even just a splash with room temperature water, works well on mature skins. Some women notice their facial skin becomes oilier as their hormone levels change – witch hazel is astringent, without being too drying and is available at most pharmacies. Any of these spritzers would be useful to cool a flush, too.

Moisture boost

Use a moisturiser on your face morning and night. They lock in moisture and form a protective barrier, which is why they work best when applied whilst your skin is still damp. There are lots to choose from – many with particular claims regarding wrinkle prevention, or even removal! Research has shown that expensive creams aren't necessarily any better than cheaper brands – all moisturisers are basically a mixture of water and oil. However, experts particularly recommend those containing peptides, retinol and antioxidants, including vitamins C and E, for ageing skin. As skin tends to be drier after the menopause, go for a richer cream designed for mature skins. If you have an oily T-zone, just apply moisturiser where you need it – on your cheeks and neck. Don't forget to moisturise your body too – especially after bathing or showering. A basic baby lotion or similar product will do the job.

Your neck has fewer fat cells and sebaceous glands, so it tends to age more quickly than your face. For a crepey neck, apply a richer moisturiser and try using patchouli or neroli oil, as recommended in chapter 6.

DIY peel

Commercial facial peels usually contain AHAs – alpha-hydroxy acids – which peel away dead skin cells to reveal the smoother, younger skin beneath. They're slightly gentler than the traditional grainy face scrub exfoliators, but do the same job. Milk, fruits and vegetables (apples, grapes, pineapples, oranges, lemons, tomatoes and cucumbers) all contain AHAs. For an easy peel, apply milk with cotton wool. Alternatively, rub a slice of your chosen fruit or vegetable over your face and neck. Tomatoes and cucumbers are moisturising. Both lemon and orange are good for oily patches and help to lighten 'liver spots'. Leave for 5 minutes and then rinse off with tepid water. Pat dry, then apply moisturiser – exfoliation improves its absorption. Caution: if you experience a stinging sensation, rinse off immediately. Face peels can also cause increased sensitivity to sunlight, so ensure you wear a sunscreen.

Anti-cellulite scrub

No matter how carefully we eat, or how active we are, many women have cellulite. Hormonal changes and ageing skin seem to be implicated. Cellulite appears when fat cells swell and push through the surrounding fibrous tissue, giving a dimpled effect. This home-made, invigorating and moisturising, anti-cellulite scrub uses items from your kitchen cupboard.

Ingredients
1 cup sea salt
1 cup ground coffee
2 tbsp olive oil

Simply mix all of the ingredients together and massage into wet skin, either in the bath or shower. Coffee has been used in this way for a number of years in tropical spas – the caffeine is believed to tone and tighten the skin and shrink fat cells.

Luscious lips

The skin on your lips is very thin and doesn't contain oil-producing sebaceous glands, so it needs a richer moisturiser for protection from the elements. Ideally, wear a lipstick or lip gloss containing an SPF of at least 15, or apply a little sunscreen under your usual lip colour. Vaseline makes a cheap but effective lip gloss cum lip balm. Honey makes a great treatment for dry, sore lips. Apply just before bed and leave on overnight.

Your lips tend to lose their fullness with age, largely due to loss of fat and collagen. To make your lips appear plumper, use light to medium lipsticks and glosses – dark shades can make them appear even thinner. Shimmery tones also give an illusion of fullness, whereas matt ones do the opposite.

Eye-q

The skin around your eyes is the thinnest on your body, so moisture evaporates more easily, which is why we tend to develop lines around our eyes before we do anywhere else. The main thing to remember is that the skin in the eye area is fragile, so avoid rubbing or scrubbing it. Dab moisturiser or eye cream in gently. Avoid very heavy creams or oils, as they can cause puffiness.

Flush-resistant make-up

If your face tends to sweat and go red when you flush, getting make-up to stay put can be a problem. The following tips may help:

- If redness is a problem, try Boots No.7 Colour Calming Make-Up Base. It's a green-tinted cream that neutralises rosy skin tones. Use it before applying make-up, or on its own.

- Tinted moisturiser looks more natural and is less likely to run than foundation.

- Use waterproof mascara, eyeliner and eyeshadow. Avoid matte eyeshadow; opt instead for sheer, shimmering shades.

- A clear gel blusher tends not to streak as much as a powder one.

Hand-y hints

Neglected hands can be an instant age giveaway. Like your neck and lips, your hands have fewer oil glands, so they're prone to drying out. To make things worse, we subject our hands to all sorts of ill-treatment every day. They're exposed to harsh soaps and hot water as well as household chemicals, which dry out the natural oils. To protect your hands wear rubber gloves when doing housework. During the winter wear gloves to shield your hands from the elements. To replace lost moisture, carry a tube of hand cream with you. Reapply frequently during the day and last thing at night. Sugar mixed with olive oil makes a great hand scrub.

Nail it

Like skin and hair, nails reflect good nutrition, or otherwise. Many of the nutrients that help to relieve menopausal symptoms promote healthy nails too. Essential fatty acids keep nails strong and supple. Isoflavones, calcium and zinc may improve nail growth and strength. Vitamin E gives strength and lustre.

External treatments can help too. Use a nail buffer regularly to boost blood flow and add gloss. Follow the manufacturer's instructions – overzealous use of the roughest edge can damage the nail. Massage hand cream or almond or olive oil into your nails and cuticles each night before bed and you'll soon notice a dramatic improvement in their condition.

49 Get heavenly hair

In a recent poll by a high street chemist, one in three women said that their hair was the most important aspect of their appearance. Unfortunately, the menopause is a time when your hair, like your skin, may reflect your body's lower oestrogen levels by becoming thinner and drier. However, with the right diet and care, it's still possible to have heavenly hair.

Hair food

Heavy bleeding during the perimenopause can cause an iron deficiency, which is often a cause of hair thinning and loss. A poor diet, lacking in protein, B vitamins and vitamin C can also play a part. To increase your iron levels eat plenty of green vegetables and some red meat, which also provides the amino acid lysine – essential for iron absorption. Eat lots of fresh fruit, especially citrus – the vitamin C they contain aids iron absorption.

A lack of zinc can also contribute to hair loss. Shellfish, green leafy vegetables, nuts and seeds are good sources. Sulphur is important for healthy hair growth and is found in onions, eggs and garlic. Include wholegrains for vitamin B complex. A lack of the B vitamin biotin is associated with hair loss and premature greying. Eggs, soya, liver, nuts and cereals are good sources. Finally, eat oily fish, nuts and seeds for omega-3 fatty acids and vitamin E to help beat dryness.

Thyroid problems can also cause hair loss. See 'Is it the Menopause?' in the introduction and details of Thyroid UK in the directory. Visit your GP if you suspect you have anaemia or a thyroid problem.

Stimulating scalp massage

This scalp massage improves hair growth and health by boosting circulation. It also doubles up as a stress reliever! Place your fingertips on each side of your head just above the ears and rotate them firmly for 30 seconds, ensuring that your scalp moves. Working towards the middle, move on to the next spot and then to the next, until you've covered the whole scalp.

Tip: use this technique whilst shampooing your hair.

Go for gloss

For glossy locks, make sure you choose the right type of shampoo for your hair type. Always condition after shampooing, concentrating on the mid-lengths and ends. Rinse well, ending with cool water. Finish off with a tiny amount of serum, to protect your hair from styling aids, prevent dryness and flyaway hair and add shine. Top stylists recommend a trim every six weeks to avoid split ends and keep hair looking its best.

Style counsel

The main point about hairstyle is to avoid getting stuck in a time warp. Aim at updating your style every few years. Nothing is more ageing than sporting the same style you had 20 years ago. Find a hair stylist you feel listens to you. Take pictures to give an idea of the look you're after. Ask for advice on which cuts will complement both your face shape and hair type.

Colour me beautiful

For many of us, grey hair is a sign of ageing that we'd rather keep hidden. The age at which you start to go grey, and how quickly, is largely genetic, but lifestyle factors such as stress and a lack of certain nutrients can play a part. If you decide to conceal your grey hairs with colour, remember going darker can be too harsh and ageing. As you age you also lose pigment from your skin, so it's best to opt for hair colour that's a shade or two lighter than your pre-grey hue.

If you decide to go grey gracefully, remember grey hair is usually coarser and drier, due to loss of pigment. It may need more conditioning and more frequent trimming to keep it looking good. Select a gentle shampoo specifically for grey hair – try Klorane Cornflower (Centaury) Shampoo for grey/white hair – to enhance natural highlights.

De-fuzz

If you begin to sprout facial hair around the time of the menopause, it's likely you're the victim of another unfortunate side effect of hormonal changes. If you grow more than is easily manageable with tweezers, your options for removal include using a facial hair bleaching cream, a depilatory cream or a home waxing kit. Electrolysis, or laser hair removal, may offer a more long-term solution, but make sure you consult a qualified practitioner or ask your GP for a referral to a suitable dermatologist.

50 Banish middle-age spread

A slower metabolism and lower oestrogen levels at menopause can lead to weight gain and a redistribution of body fat, as the body tries to hang on to oestrogen-producing fat cells by storing them round the middle – resulting in a thicker waist. Carrying too much fat around your middle increases the risk of serious health problems such as heart disease, high blood pressure, stroke and diabetes. If you're postmenopausal, carrying excess weight increases your risk of breast cancer by 50 per cent. Below are some tips to help you beat middle-age spread.

Check your waist size

A waist size of 80 cm indicates increased risk. A waist measurement of 88 cm or above means you're at a high risk of ill-health. To measure your waist, place a tape measure around the narrowest point between your lower ribs and your hips.

Calculate your BMI

Calculating your body mass index (BMI) can also help you determine whether you're a healthy weight. Do this by multiplying your height in metres, by your height in metres. Now divide your weight in kilos by this figure.

For example, if you're 1.6 metres tall and weigh 65 kg:
1.6 x 1.6 = 2.56
65 / 2.56 = 25.39

A BMI of 18.5–24.9 indicates a healthy weight. Below 18.5 is classed as underweight, whilst 25–29.9 is deemed overweight. A BMI of 30–39.9 indicates obesity and 40 and above signifies morbid obesity. Basically, if you have a BMI of 25 or over, you should consider losing weight. But bear in mind your BMI is only a guide – if you're quite muscular, with little fat, you could still have a high BMI as it measures weight rather than fat in relation to height.

Go for low GI foods

For a healthy way of eating that will help you lose excess pounds – especially around your middle – choose foods with a low glycaemic index. The glycaemic index (GI) is a measure of how quickly a food raises the level of sugar in the blood.

Carbohydrates with a high GI are easily broken down into glucose, causing your blood sugar to rise rapidly and then fall just as quickly. Refined foods like white bread, pastries, sugary drinks and sweets tend to have a high GI. Carbohydrates with a low GI take longer to digest and cause your blood glucose to rise slowly and steadily, helping you feel full for longer and therefore eat less. Unrefined foods, including multigrain bread, porridge, sweet potatoes, wholewheat pasta and brown rice have a low GI. Because they release glucose slowly into the bloodstream, these foods may reduce the risk of type 2 diabetes. It's thought that the fibre in these foods slows down glucose absorption. Fibre helps weight loss in other ways – it fills you up more quickly, so you eat less. Also, your body burns fat when it breaks down fibre.

Eat plenty of fruit and vegetables, dairy products, including yogurt, milk and cheese, and small portions of nuts, fish and lean meat. Leave the skins on potatoes to lower their GI – eating potatoes without the skin allows the glucose to be digested more rapidly. Boiled new potatoes with their skins left on have the lowest GI. Such a diet will enable you to lose weight, whilst providing the balance of nutrients needed for good health.

Tip: sprinkling a little vinegar over your meals can help to slow down the rate of absorption of glucose from food.

Soy good

Including soya-based foods and drinks in your diet may help you avoid weight gain around the middle. A recent study showed that a group of women who drank a soya-based shake each day gained less fat on their stomachs than a group who didn't. Researchers believed the phytoestrogens in the soya affected fat metabolism.

Dairy maid

We've already seen in chapter 4 that dairy foods provide calcium, which helps ease menopausal symptoms and prevent osteoporosis. But did you know that calcium also helps weight loss – especially around the middle?

In a recent American study a group of overweight people eating a diet containing 1,200 mg of calcium from dairy foods lost 70 per cent more weight and three times the fat from their waists, than a group eating no dairy foods, but identical calories, fat, carbohydrate and protein. It seems that calcium reduces the amount of fat we absorb from foods, whilst speeding up our metabolism.

Eat protein

Studies show that eating protein at each meal can help you lose weight. When eaten with carbohydrates, protein makes you feel fuller for longer, because it slows down the rate glucose is released into the bloodstream, so you're likely to eat less.

Protein also boosts the metabolism, enabling you to burn more calories. This is especially useful after the menopause, when the metabolism tends to slow down. It's thought the body burns about one third of the calories from protein foods when breaking them down. It also seems to prompt the body to burn fat for energy. As animal proteins are high in saturated fats, choose oily and white fish, low-fat dairy foods, soya and lean meats. Also, don't eat more than the recommended handful at each meal, as experts warn that high protein diets, such as the Atkins Diet, can lead to kidney problems and osteoporosis.

Breakfast well

Research shows that eating breakfast helps weight management. Breakfast eaters tend not to eat as much during the day – probably because their blood sugar remains steadier. A recent study of a group of 40- to 75-year-old men and women found that those eating one fifth to a half of their calories at breakfast gained less weight than those who skipped it, or ate very little. Researchers concluded that eating breakfast boosts the metabolism, whereas going without encourages the body to go into starvation mode and store fat.

Vive la France!

Taking time to enjoy preparing, cooking and eating your food, rather than simply grabbing a ready meal, seems to help weight control. French women in particular have a reputation for enjoying their food, whilst remaining slim and healthy. The French generally avoid snacking and take the time to prepare meals from fresh ingredients and eat slowly, savouring their food. They also tend to make mealtimes more of an occasion, sitting at the table rather than in front of the TV. Whilst they might eat bread and chocolate, they focus on flavour and quality, rather than quantity, avoiding junk foods. So they're likely to choose a little freshly baked bread and a couple of squares of plain, cocoa rich chocolate, rather than stodgy sliced bread and over-sweet milk chocolate. They also eat lots of fruit and vegetables and dairy products. Their philosophy seems to be, enjoy healthy, good-quality food and eat what you fancy – just in small amounts. If you want to lose weight, perhaps developing a French attitude towards food could help.

Easy portion size guide

To follow the example of the French, you need to control your portion sizes. Even if you choose healthy foods, if you eat too much of them you'll put on weight. Here's an easy guide:

- Carbohydrate foods (pasta, potatoes and rice): two handfuls Vegetables/salad: two or more handfuls
- Protein foods (meat, eggs and fish): one handful
- Cheese: one matchbox-sized piece
- Nuts: one small handful
- Fats and oils: one tablespoon or less

Balanced plate

For a balanced meal, one third should be carbohydrates, one third vegetables or fruit, one sixth a protein food (meat, fish or a meat alternative like soya mince) and one sixth dairy. Women need about 500 calories a day fewer than men, so serve yourself smaller portions – about a fifth less – than your partner's.

Fats and weight

When it comes to weight, fats get a bad press and low-fat diets are viewed as the best way to lose weight. Whilst fat is relatively high in calories – 1 g contains 9 calories, whereas 1 g of carbohydrate or protein contains 4 calories – it's vital for various bodily functions. Fats also make food more satisfying and keep you full for longer by slowing down the rate at which glucose is absorbed, so they can actually help you manage your weight.

However, it's important to restrict the amount of fats you eat to avoid weight gain, and to avoid the fats which are detrimental to health. Choose the healthier polyunsaturated (omega-3 and omega-6) and monounsaturated (omega-9) fats discussed in chapter 4, instead.

Remember, foods rich in these fats include oily fish, egg yolks, nuts, seeds, wholegrains, dark green leafy vegetables and oils such as sunflower and olive. Nutritionists recommend no more than a third of our daily energy intake should come from fats. This is the equivalent of about 75 g for women, of which no more than 20 g should be saturated fat.

Cut down on unhealthy fats

Saturated fats, also known as hard fats, are mainly found in animal products such as red meat, butter and full-fat dairy foods like cheese and milk. All saturated fats used to get a bad press, but recent research suggests that those found in meat and dairy foods may help with weight management by keeping us fuller for longer and may have other health benefits. It's now thought that saturated fats found in processed meats such as sausages, beefburgers and bacon are more harmful and best avoided due to their link with an increased risk of heart disease and atherosclerosis (hardening of the arteries). They may also be linked to some cancers, such as breast cancer.

Trans-fatty acids, or trans-fats, are mainly found in processed foods and are usually listed on the packaging as 'hydrogenated' or 'partially hydrogenated' vegetable oil/fat. Manufacturers use them to extend the shelf life of their products. They're formed when liquid vegetable oils are turned into solid fats, through a process called hydrogenation. Trans-fats may lead to weight gain – especially around the middle. A six-year study showed that a group of monkeys whose diet contained trans-fats gained over three times as much weight as monkeys whose diets contained monounsaturated fats. They also carried around a third more fat on their tummies.

To reduce your intake of unhealthy fats:

- Avoid eating processed meats – go for good-quality fresh meats instead.

- Grill, bake, poach, steam and microwave instead of frying or roasting.

- Skim off any fat that rises to the top during cooking.

- Avoid processed foods with hydrogenated fat and trans-fatty acids in the ingredients list.

- Use herbs and strong condiments to add flavour to foods instead of high-fat sauces – try mustard, soy sauce and balsamic or white wine vinegar.

Put an end to comfort eating

The low mood some women experience during the peri- and postmenopause can lead to comfort eating, which can in turn lead to weight gain. If you often eat for emotional reasons rather than true hunger, you need to change your behaviour around food, whilst dealing with the underlying issues. Make it a rule that you only eat in response to true (stomach) hunger rather than emotional (mouth) hunger. If, like many women, you've dieted and binged for years, you may find it hard to recognise when you're hungry. Notice how your body signals it needs food. For some people hunger makes itself known by contractions and gurgling in the stomach; others notice similar sensations in the chest or throat.

Do something new

Meanwhile, explore the reasons why you're comfort eating and then look at ways of dealing with them. For example, if you're feeling depressed and lonely, perhaps because your children have left home, consider ways of widening your social circle. Now is a good time to take up a new interest or hobby that could lead to new friendships, for example yoga, salsa dancing, a cookery or art class – do whatever interests you. Doing new things has been shown to encourage weight loss, because it helps to divert your mental focus away from food.

Break the cycle

Stress can also lead to comfort eating – especially of fatty and sugary foods, which seem to act as an antidote to stress hormones and induce feelings of calm. If you tend to overeat when stressed, it's important to break the cycle by finding other ways to deal with tension. For example, after a stressful day at work, instead of reaching for the biscuit tin have a soak in a warm bath with a relaxing, aromatic oil, such as lavender or camomile. Chapter 1 offers more tips on lifting depression and relieving stress. See also the section on foods that boost mood in chapter 4. Remember, being active and getting out in the daylight boost your levels of the 'happy hormone' serotonin, which is also involved in appetite control.

Fit in fitness

Exercise is not only vital for good health, it's also key to weight control. Being physically active aids weight loss by burning calories and speeding up the metabolism. Current recommendations suggest we should undertake moderate activity, like walking, at least 30 minutes a day, five times a week. To lose weight, aim at increasing this to 60 minutes daily, five times a week.

Many people find visiting the gym difficult to keep up with, but there are plenty of simple ways of increasing the amount of physical activity you do in your everyday life.

In chapter 5 we looked at how exercise, including walking, can help beat many menopausal symptoms, such as hot flushes, depression and osteoporosis, and how easy it is to develop the habit of walking more. Walking is also a great way to burn calories and lose weight.

Domestic goddess

Housework and gardening are also good forms of exercise which burn calories and build fitness. Shopping, hanging out washing on the clothes line and cleaning windows all burn calories and help tone muscles.

Tip: being active, even for just a few minutes, several times a day, stimulates the body to produce more fat-busting enzymes than if you only exercise once.

Recipes

This section contains recipes based on the dietary recommendations outlined in chapter 4.

Hummus

In this recipe the chickpeas provide plant oestrogens and soluble fibre.

Ingredients

200 g canned chickpeas
1 tbsp tahini (sesame seed paste) – optional
2 cloves garlic (or more to taste)
1 tsp ground cumin
1 lemon, squeezed
A tiny sprinkle of salt
Black pepper

Method

1. Drain and rinse the chickpeas and blend to a coarse paste.
2. Add the tahini, garlic, cumin and lemon juice and blend again.
3. Season to taste.
4. Serve with warm pitta bread and salad, or use as a dip with vegetable crudités.

Mixed bean salad (serves two)

In this recipe, the beans and vegetables provide plant oestrogens and soluble fibre. The red pepper provides the antioxidant vitamins A and C.

Ingredients
400 g can of mixed beans
1 stick of celery
Half a red onion, finely chopped
1 red pepper, finely chopped
1 medium tomato
1 tbsp fresh basil

Dressing
2 tbsp olive oil
2 tbsp balsamic vinegar
1 clove garlic, crushed

Method
1. Rinse the beans in cold water and drain. Then place in a bowl.
2. Add salad vegetables and basil and mix together.
3. Blend together dressing ingredients and combine with beans and vegetables.
4. Place in refrigerator to chill.
5. Serve with crusty brown bread.

Soya milk smoothie

In this recipe, the soya milk provides isoflavones, protein and calcium.

Ingredients

1 large banana
2–3 handfuls of fruit
285 ml of soya milk
Runny honey (optional)
Cinnamon (optional)

Method

1. Place the banana and your chosen fruit into a blender.
2. Blend for 30 seconds.
3. Add the soya milk and honey to taste.
4. Blend again to milkshake consistency.
5. Sprinkle with cinnamon and serve.

HRT cake

This cake provides a rich source of a range of phytoestrogens, vitamin E and soluble and insoluble fibre.

Ingredients

100 g soya flour
100 g wholewheat flour
100 g porridge oats
100 g linseeds
50 g sunflower seeds
50 g sesame seeds
50 g flaked almonds/walnut pieces
2 pieces chopped stem ginger
200 g raisins/sultanas
3 g nutmeg
3 g cinnamon

3 g ground ginger

Approx. 500 ml soya milk

1 tbsp malt extract

3 tbsp chopped dried apricots/dates/prunes/cranberries

Method

1. Place the dry ingredients in a large bowl and mix well.
2. Next add the soya milk and malt extract. Mix well and leave for 30 minutes. If the mixture is too firm, add more soya milk.
3. Spoon the mix into two lightly oiled loaf tins, lined with greaseproof paper.
4. Bake in an oven at 190°C/375°F for around 75 minutes, or until cooked right through. Test with a skewer – it should come out clean.
5. Turn out and cool on a wire rack.
6. Serve in thick slices with a vegetable margarine or soya spread.

> **Tip**
>
> If you need more sweetness, try it with a little honey.

Menopause muffins (makes 12)

These contain beetroot and soya milk, which are rich in phytoestrogens. Beetroot also contains nitrates, which help to widen the blood vessels and boost the circulation – this may help to ease hot flushes. The sunflower seeds also provide plant oestrogens and vitamin E.

Ingredients

150 g wholemeal flour
150 g rolled oats
1¼ tsp baking powder
½ tsp baking soda
Pinch of salt
1 tsp ground cinnamon
1 tsp mixed spice
1 ripe banana
2 medium raw beetroots, peeled and finely grated
100 ml rapeseed oil
2 tbsp honey
2 eggs, beaten
250 ml soya milk
50 g raisins
50 g sunflower seeds

Method

1. Preheat oven to 190°C/375°F.
2. Line a twelve-hole muffin tin with paper muffin cases.
3. Mix the dry ingredients in a large bowl.
4. In a separate bowl, mash the banana. Add grated beetroot, oil, honey, eggs and soya milk, and mix.
5. Add to the dry ingredients and mix well before adding raisins and sunflower seeds.
6. Share the mixture out equally among the muffin cases.
7. Bake for 20–25 minutes until golden and the tip of inserted knife/skewer comes out clean.
8. Cool on a wire rack and store in an airtight container for up to five days.

Warm lentil salad (serves four)

The lentils provide plant lignans and coumestans, as well as both soluble and insoluble fibre.

Ingredients
225 g puy, green or brown lentils
2 red peppers
200 g goat's cheese
2 tbsp balsamic vinegar
4 tbsp olive oil
50 g sun-dried tomatoes

Method
1. Add 275 ml of boiling water to the lentils and then cook over a low heat for about 40 minutes.
2. Slice and chargrill the red peppers 10 minutes before they're ready.
3. Slice the goat's cheese and place on a baking tray under the grill until slightly melted.
4. Place the drained lentils in a warmed serving bowl.
5. Mix together the balsamic vinegar and olive oil and pour over.
6. Stir in the chargrilled peppers and sun-dried tomatoes.
7. Place the goat's cheese on top.
8. Serve immediately.

Tofu, vegetable and bean sprout stir-fry (serves two)

In this recipe the tofu and beansprouts provide isoflavones and coumestans.

Ingredients
2 tbsp olive oil
2 cloves garlic
2 carrots
1 red pepper
1 green pepper
4 spring onions
1 pack of marinated tofu pieces
Soy sauce to taste
1 small bag of bean sprouts

Method
1. Slice the vegetables into thin strips. Peel and crush the garlic.
2. Heat the olive oil in a wok and stir-fry the vegetables and garlic for 3 to 4 minutes.
3. Add the tofu and soy sauce and heat through.
4. Add the bean sprouts and cook for a further couple of minutes – until they are tender but still crisp.
5. Serve immediately.

Avocado dip (serves two to four)

Avocados are rich in monounsaturated fats, fibre and antioxidants.

Ingredients
1 avocado
1 garlic clove, crushed
Half a fresh green chilli, finely chopped
Juice of half a lemon/1 lime
Black pepper to taste

Method
Simply blend the ingredients together and serve with warm mini pitta breads and carrots, or celery cut into dipping-sized batons.

Prostaglandins – hormone-like chemicals produced in the body to create a number of effects, including the stimulation of contractions in the uterus and other smooth muscle.

Receptors – proteins on the surface of cells designed to bind with and react to specific substances in the body, e.g. hormones and insulin.

Jargon Buster

Acetylcholine – chemical involved in learning and memory.

Adaptogen – substance which helps the body adapt to and deal with stress.

Amino acids – organic acids which form the building blocks of proteins.

Androgen – a male hormone.

Anti-oestrogenic – suppressing or neutralising the action of oestrogen.

Atherosclerosis – narrowing of the arteries, caused by fatty deposits.

Atrophy – wasting of body organ, or tissue, through various causes, including hormonal changes.

Beta-carotene – the plant form of vitamin A, found in orange or green coloured fruits and vegetables, e.g. oranges, carrots and green vegetables. An antioxidant.

Bioflavonoids – substances found in fruits such as lemons, blackcurrants and plums, which improve the function of vitamin C.

Collagen – structural protein found in connective tissues, including the skin and bones.

Cortisol – hormone produced by the adrenal glands.

Coumestans – plant oestrogens found mainly in bean sprouts.

Free radicals – substances produced by normal chemical reactions in the body and linked to cell damage.

FSH – stands for follicle-stimulating hormone, which is produced by the pituitary gland and triggers the ripening of the follicles in the ovary. This in turn stimulates the ovaries to produce oestrogen.

GABA – stands for Gamma-aminobutyric acid, an amino acid that acts as a chemical messenger in the brain, spinal cord, heart, lungs and kidneys, telling the body to slow down.

GI – stands for glycaemic index, a ranking of foods according to the effect they have on blood sugar levels.

Hormones – chemicals produced by glands to carry messages to various organs in the body.

Isoflavones – plant oestrogens found mainly in soya and other legumes.

Libido – sex drive.

Lignans – plant oestrogens found in cereals, fruits, vegetables and seeds.

Melatonin – hormone produced by the pineal gland in the brain which regulates sleep.

Metabolism – physical and chemical processes by which substances are broken down into energy or produced for use in the body.

Oestrogen – the collective term for three female hormones: oestradiol, oestriol and oestrone. Produced mainly by the ovaries, but also by the adrenal glands and fat cells.

Oestrogenic – having an action that's similar to that of oestrogen.

Phytochemicals – chemicals which occur naturally in plants and are thought to be beneficial to health.

Phytoestrogens – plant hormones from which the body produces substances that have a similar effect on the body as oestrogen.

Phytonutrients – see Phytochemicals.

Prebiotics – natural indigestible starches which feed and encourage the growth of existing good bacteria in the gut.

Precursor – a substance used by the body to produce another substance.

Probiotics – literally means 'for life'. Beneficial bacteria found in foods such as natural yogurt, which are thought to aid digestion and boost the immune system.

Progesterone – literal meaning is 'for pregnancy'. Female hormone involved in the preparation of the womb for pregnancy.

Prostaglandins – are hormones produced at sites of tissue damage or infection, where they cause inflammation, pain and fever as part of the healing process.

Receptor – a specialised cell that responds to sensory stimuli, e.g. skin receptors respond to touch and pressure. Also a structure found on or within a cell that binds to a hormone, or other chemical substance.

Selenium – a trace mineral essential to the body.

Serotonin – a chemical involved in various bodily functions, including mood, appetite, sleep and sensory perception.

Triglycerides – fats produced in the liver from foods eaten and from internal fat, either for energy or storage.

Tryptophan – amino acid that is used by the body to make mood-enhancing serotonin.

Useful Products

The following products may help to ease menopausal symptoms. The author doesn't endorse or recommend any particular product and this list is by no means exhaustive.

Acupressure For Menopause App
A free app with images and video clips that show traditional Chinese massage points for the relief of menopausal symptoms.
 Website: www.windowsphone.com

Australian Bush Flower Essences
These are similar to Bach Flower Remedies but, as the name implies, are based on Australian plants and contain a mixture of plant essences to deal with particular conditions. Woman Essence and Woman Cream are recommended during the menopause to promote hormonal balance, balanced moods and calm.
 Website: www.flowersense.co.uk

Boots Ginkgo Biloba 120 mg
Tablets containing ginkgo biloba. Free from artificial colours, flavours and preservatives. Gluten and lactose free. Suitable for vegetarians.
 Website: www.boots.com

Boots Starflower Oil 1,000 mg
Capsules containing gamma linolenic acid (GLA) and vitamin E. Free from artificial colours, flavours and preservatives. Gluten and lactose free. Suitable for vegetarians.
 Website: www.boots.com

The Chillow

A foam pillow that stays cool once you have activated it by filling with cold tap water – ideal to help you deal with hot flushes and night sweats.

Website: www.chillow.co.uk

The Cobber Body Cooling Neck Wrap

A scarf which lowers your body temperature by cooling the carotid arteries in your neck. Made from polyester and cotton, it contains poly-crystals which, once activated by soaking in cool water, provide an evaporative cooling system. It's available in various colours and designs and it's ideal for relieving flushes, both indoors and when you're out and about.

Website: www.nomadtravel.co.uk

The Diet Plate

A plate designed to help you control your portion sizes and eat correctly balanced meals, thus aiding weight control.

Website: www.thedietplate.com

Eurovital Melatonin

Capsules containing 3 mg of melatonin.

Website: www.biovea.net/UK

Hand-held, battery-operated fan

These have soft, flexible, blades. It's portable and also converts to a free-standing tabletop fan, so it's ideal for use at the office.

Website: www.livingiseasy.co.uk

LadyCare

A discreet magnetic device that you attach to your underwear. In a trial of the product involving over 500 women, many reported a reduction in symptoms such as hot flushes, irritability, vaginal dryness and weight gain. Available in selected supermarkets and pharmacies or online.

Website: www.ladycare-uk.com

Magicool

A cooling, microfine, bacteria-free spray that self-chills and doesn't need refrigeration. Available from most high street chemists and online.

Website: www.expresschemist.co.uk

Menosan Sage Drops

A tincture of organically grown sage leaves. The recommended dose is 15–20 drops in a little water three times daily initially and then once a day to maintain the benefits.

Website: www.avogel.co.uk

Multi-Gyn gel

A soothing and moisturising natural gel for the treatment of vaginal dryness and atrophy, containing aloe, camomile, calendula, tea tree and rosemary.

Website: www.multi-gyn.com

Novogen Menopause Test

Detects the level of follicle-stimulating hormone (FSH) in the urine. Elevated levels of FSH are a clear indication of the body's transition to menopause. Manufacturer claims 99 per cent accuracy. Note: test needs to be repeated after seven days.

Website: www.pharmacy2u.co.uk

Physicool Rapid Cooling Mist

An alcohol-based mist which has a calming, cooling effect as it evaporates from warm skin.

Website: www.cooling-mist.co.uk

Rosewater

Distilled from organic rose petals. Spray it on your face and neck during a hot flush for its cooling, astringent effect and the uplifting aroma of rose essence. It's also a natural toner and helps to reduce fine lines. Can be diluted in water and drunk or used in cooking.

Website: www.pukkaherbs.com

Replens

A hormone-free vaginal moisturising gel clinically proven to relieve vaginal atrophy and dryness. Available on prescription from your GP and over the counter at pharmacies.

Website: www.boots.com

Vielle Menopause Home Test Kit

A one-step test claimed to be 98 per cent accurate and to give a result in 3 minutes. Remember, though, that FSH levels can fluctuate and repeating the test may give a more accurate picture. Available in some supermarkets and independent pharmacies and online.

Website: www.stressnomore.co.uk

Helpful Books

Glenville, Marilyn, *Healthy Eating for the Menopause* (new revised edition 2015, Kyle Books) – contains over 100 recipes based on foods rich in phytoestrogens, essential fatty acids and antioxidants.

Greer, Germaine, *The Change: Women, ageing and the menopause* (1993, Ballantine Books) – although this is now a fairly old title, it's still a great read to help you come to terms with the psychological, physical and social aspects of the menopause.

MacGregor, Anne, *Is HRT Right For You?* (2003, Sheldon Press) – written by a doctor with a special interest in women's hormones, this is a comprehensive and balanced guide on the risks and benefits of HRT, with information on the various HRT products.

Parker-Pope, Tara, *HRT – Everything you need to know to: untangle the controversy, understand your options and make your own choices* (2007, Rodale International Ltd) – this book helps you to separate HRT fact from HRT fiction.

Directory

Bladder and Bowel Foundation

Formerly known as Incontact and the Continence Foundation, the UK's leading charity providing information and support for people with bladder and bowel disorders – including IBS – their carers, families and healthcare professionals.

Website: www.bladderandbowelfoundation.org

Breast Cancer Care

Offers free information about breast health and breast cancer, and practical assistance and emotional support to anyone affected by breast cancer.

Helpline: 0808 800 6000

Website: www.breastcancercare.org.uk

British Acupuncture Council

The British Acupuncture Council (BAcC) is the leading self-regulatory body for the practice of traditional acupuncture in the UK. The website offers fact sheets about acupuncture, as well as a directory of registered traditional acupuncturists. All BAcC members have undergone degree-level training in traditional acupuncture, Chinese medicine and Western biomedical sciences, including anatomy, physiology and pathology, and must comply with the BAcC Code of Safe Practice and Code of Professional Conduct.

Website: www.acupuncture.org.uk

The British Heart Foundation

A charity offering advice and information to help you keep your heart healthy. Also offers support and resources to heart patients and their families.

Heart helpline: 0300 330 3311
Website: www.bhf.org.uk

The British Menopause Society

A registered charity which aims to increase awareness of menopausal healthcare issues.

Website: www.thebms.org.uk

Cancer Research UK

The world's leading independent organisation dedicated to cancer research. Provides cancer information and support.

Website: www.cancerresearchuk.org

Citizen's Advice Bureau

Helps people resolve their legal, financial, emotional and other problems by providing free, independent and confidential advice. Visit the website for online advice and contact details for your local CAB.

Website: www.citizensadvice.org.uk

Cruse Bereavement Care

Promotes the well-being of bereaved people and helps them to understand their grief and cope with their loss. Provides support and offers information, advice, education and training services.

Helpline: 0844 477 9400
Email: helpline@cruse.org.uk
Website: www.cruse.org.uk

The Daisy Network

A support group for women who have gone through the menopause before the age of 45.

Website: www.daisynetwork.org.uk

Drinkaware

A UK charity that works with the medical community, third-sector organisations, the government and the drinks industry to reduce alcohol misuse and harm in the UK. It provides evidence-based information about alcohol.

Website: www.drinkaware.co.uk

Elderly Parents

Organisation that offers free, impartial advice about health, home, travel, finance and wills to those responsible for the welfare of elderly parents or relatives.

Website: www.elderlyparents.org.uk

Food and Mood

Explores the relationship between what you eat and how you feel and offers tips on how to incorporate healthy eating into your life.

Website: www.mind.org.uk/foodandmood

The Happiness Project

Founded by psychologist Dr Robert Holden. Aims to help people find happiness by changing the way they think. Offers courses in happiness and positivity. The website includes an Inspiration Room with inspiring quotes, and articles, and an online happiness test.

Website: www.robertholden.org

Medicines and Healthcare products Regulatory Agency (MHRA)

A government agency responsible for ensuring that medicines and medical devices work and are acceptably safe. The website includes a section on the safety of herbal medicines and a full list of herbal medicines granted a traditional herbal registration (THR).

Website: www.mhra.gov.uk

Menopause Matters

An independent, clinician-led website aiming to provide up-to-date, accurate information about the menopause and treatment options.

Website: www.menopausematters.co.uk

Mind

A national charity for emotional and mental health problems. Offers advice online and through a network of local Mind associations which offer counselling, befriending, drop-in sessions, etc. The charity also provides two confidential mental health information services, the Mind Infoline and the Legal Advice Service.

Mind Infoline: 0300 123 3393 – 9 a.m. to 6 p.m., Monday to Friday, (except for bank holidays)

Text Infoline: 86463

Email: info@mind.org.uk

Website: www.mind.org.uk

National Debtline

Offers free confidential and independent advice on how to deal with debt problems. The website offers useful resources to help you deal with debt, including a four-step self-help guide, an interactive debt advice tool and an online budget form.

Freephone: 0808 808 4000 (Monday to Friday, 9 a.m. to 9 p.m., Saturday, 9.30 a.m. to 1 p.m.)

Website: www.nationaldebtline.co.uk

The National Osteoporosis Society (NOS)

The only UK-wide charity dedicated to improving the diagnosis, prevention and treatment of osteoporosis and fragility fractures. Provides a helpline staffed by nurses experienced in osteoporosis and bone health, a network of support groups and an online discussion forum.

Helpline: 0808 800 0035

Website: www.nos.org.uk

Natural by Nature Oils

A company offering a wide range of high-quality essential oils and aromatherapy advice.

Telephone: 01582 840 848

Website: www.naturalbynature.co.uk

NHS Choices

An NHS website that aims to help you make choices about your health, from how to cope with the menopause to decisions about your lifestyle, such as smoking, drinking and exercise. There is also a link to the Mumsnet NHS Choices forum on menopause.

Website: www.nhs.uk

Osteoporosis Advice

A website offering information about osteoporosis, from publicly available material.

Website: www.osteoporosistreatment.co.uk

Power Surge

An American website that describes itself as 'a warm and caring community for women in menopause'.

Website: www.power-surge.com

The Princess Royal Trust for Carers

A voluntary organisation that provides information, advice and support to carers through an interactive website and local support groups.

Website: www.carers.org

Relate

With 2,500 professionally trained counsellors, Relate is the UK's largest provider of relationship counselling and sex therapy. Offers counselling, sex therapy and relationship education to support couple and family relationships throughout life. Visit the website to find your nearest Relate, to consult a counsellor by email or to talk to a counsellor online via live chat. Alternatively, you can arrange counselling by telephone.

Website: www.relate.org.uk

Samaritans

Offers confidential non-judgemental emotional support, 24 hours a day, to people experiencing feelings of distress or despair, including those that could lead to suicide. This service is available over the telephone, by email, by letter or face-to-face.

Address: Freepost RSRB-KKBY-CYJK, PO Box 9090, Stirling, FK8 2SA
Telephone: 116 123
Email: jo@samaritans.org
Website: www.samaritans.org

Smokefree

An NHS website offering advice and support to help quit smoking. You can choose from a range of support options, including your local stop-smoking service, as well as email, text and online chat support services.

Smokefree national helpline: 0300 123 1044
Website: www.nhs.uk/smokefree

Thyroid UK

An organisation that campaigns for and provides information and support to those with thyroid disorders.

Website: www.thyroiduk.org.uk

Tisserand Aromatherapy

Offer a wide range of good-quality essential oils.

Website: www.tisserand.com

Walking for Health

England's largest network of health walk schemes, helping people across the country lead a more active life.

Website: www.walkingforhealth.org.uk

Women's Health Concern

An independent service run by the British Menopause Society. Offers women health, well-being and lifestyle advice online, as well as by email and via a telephone advisory service (donations/fees apply).

Website: www.womens-health-concern.org

PERSONAL HEALTH GUIDES

IBS

A self-help guide to feeling better

Wendy Green

Foreword by Dr Nick Read,
chair of The IBS Network

IBS
A self-help guide to feeling better

Wendy Green

£8.99
Paperback
ISBN: 978-1-84953-807-7

In this easy-to-follow book, Wendy Green explains how food intolerances, gut infections and bacterial imbalance, and stress and hormones contribute to IBS and offers practical advice and a holistic approach to help you deal with the symptoms, including simple dietary and lifestyle changes, and DIY complementary therapies. Find out 50 things you can do today to help you cope with IBS, including:

- ▶ Identify your IBS triggers and learn how to manage them
- ▶ Choose beneficial foods and supplements
- ▶ Manage stress and relax to reduce flare-ups
- ▶ Discover practical tips for living with IBS
- ▶ Adopt preventative strategies
- ▶ Find helpful organisations and products

Anxiety

A self-help guide to feeling better

Wendy Green

Foreword by Joanne Sale, senior lecturer in
mental health, University of Bedfordshire

Anxiety
A self-help guide to feeling better

Wendy Green

£8.99
Paperback
ISBN: 978-1-84953-822-0

In this easy-to-follow book, Wendy Green explains how psychological, genetic and dietary factors can contribute to anxiety and offers practical advice and a holistic approach to help you deal with the symptoms, including simple dietary and lifestyle changes and DIY complementary therapies. Find out 50 things you can do today, including:

- ► Replace negative thoughts and behaviour with positive thoughts and behaviour
- ► Manage stress and relax to reduce symptoms
- ► Choose beneficial foods and supplements
- ► Find helpful organisations and products

Migraines

A self-help guide to feeling better

Wendy Green

Foreword by Professor Anne MacGregor, specialist in headache and women's health, and honorary professor at the Centre for Neuroscience and Trauma

Migraines
A self-help guide to feeling better

Wendy Green

£8.99
Paperback
ISBN: 978-1-84953-808-4

Do you suffer from severe headaches, sometimes with nausea and visual impairment? Can these headaches last for up to a day or longer at a time? If so, you could be experiencing migraines. In this easy-to-follow book, Wendy Green explains how dietary, psychological and environmental factors can cause migraines, and offers practical advice and a holistic approach to help you manage them. Find out 50 things you can do today to help you cope with migraines, including:

- ▶ **Identify your migraine triggers and learn how to manage them**
- ▶ **Choose beneficial foods and supplements**
- ▶ **Learn how to adapt your home and work environments**
- ▶ **Discover how to treat children and teenagers with the condition**
- ▶ **Find helpful organisations and products**

Have you enjoyed this book?
If so, why not write a review on your favourite website?

If you're interested in finding out more about our books, find us on Facebook at **Summersdale Publishers** and follow us on Twitter at **@Summersdale**.

Thanks very much for buying this Summersdale book.

www.summersdale.com